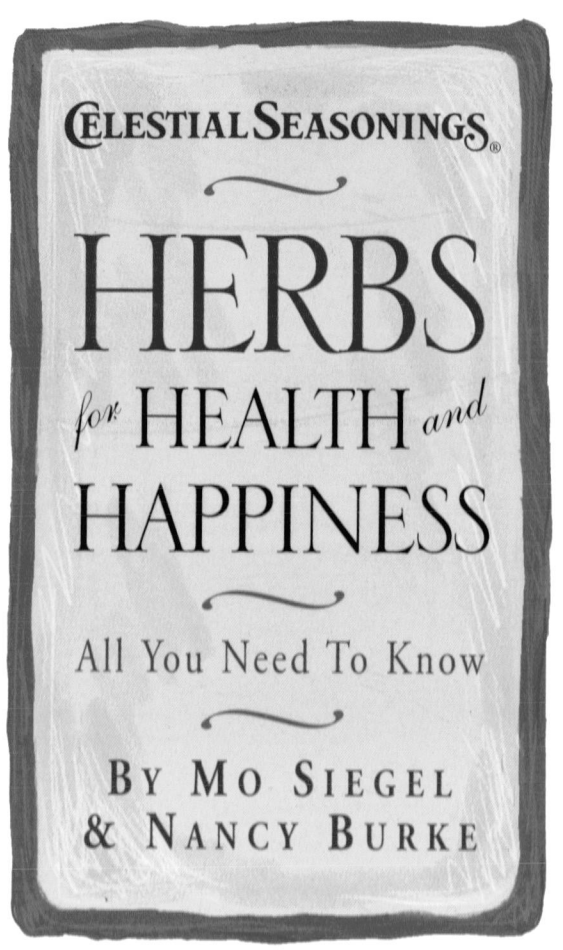

CELESTIAL SEASONINGS®

HERBS
for HEALTH *and*
HAPPINESS

All You Need To Know

BY MO SIEGEL
& NANCY BURKE

TIME
LIFE
BOOKS

ALEXANDRIA, VIRGINIA

TIME® LIFE BOOKS

Time-Life Books is a division of Time Life Inc.
TIME LIFE INC.
President and CEO: George Artandi

TIME-LIFE CUSTOM PUBLISHING

Vice President and Publisher	Terry Newell
Vice President of Sales and Marketing	Neil Levin
Director of Acquisitions and Editorial Resources	Jennifer Pearce
Editor	Linda Bellamy
Director of Creative Services	Laura McNeill
Technical Specialist	Monika Lynde
Production Manager	Carolyn Bounds
Quality Assurance Manager	James D. King

Produced by nSight Inc., Cambridge, Massachusetts. Cover design by Universal Communications, Inc. Text design by Suzanne Sarto and Joanna Zito. Illustrations by Anne Crosse.

First printing. Printed in China
TIME-LIFE is a trademark of Time Warner Inc. and affiliated companies.

Library of Congress Cataloging-in-Publication Data
Siegel, Mo.
    Celestial Seasonings' herbs for health and happiness: all you need to know/by Mo Siegel and Nancy Burke.
        p. cm.
    Includes index.
    ISBN 0-7370-0051-1 (softcover: alk paper)
    1. Herbs--Therapeutic use. I. Title: Herbs for health and happiness.
    II. Burke, Nancy, 1949- III. Celestial Seasonings (Firm) IV. Title.

RM666.H33S54 1999   99-038591
615'.321--dc21

Books produced by Time-Life Custom Publishing are available at a special bulk discount for promotional and premium use. Custom adaptations can also be created to meet your specific marketing goals. Call 1-800-323-5255.

NOTE: The medical conditions and treatment options offered in this book should be considered as reference sources only. They are not intended to substitute for a qualified medical practitioner's diagnosis, advice, treatment, and prescribed medication. Always consult your physician or a qualified practitioner for proper medical care. Before using any herb or natural medicine mentioned in this book, read any "cautions" that accompany the discussion of the herb in question and consult your practitioner or the product's packaging for any warnings, cautions, and contraindications. Remember: Herbal remedies are not as strictly regulated as drugs.

Acknowledgments

My deepest thanks go to God for the wonders of nature. My life has been continuously blessed by constant hikes in the wilderness where an abundance of wild herbs grace the towering Rocky Mountains.

My warmest thanks go to all the naturalists, botanists, herbalists, and health advocates who shaped my hobbies of hiking and herbs into a useful career.

And special thanks to all the fine people who poured their hearts and souls into making Celestial Seasonings America's favorite herb company.

Super thanks to Sherry Dickerson, my most able and dedicated assistant.

Thanks to Nancy Burke for her writing in this book, to Joanna Zito and Suzanne Sarto for the book design, to Ellen Kresky for her coordination, to Kerin Franklin for her botanical science, to Kate Hartson and Linda Bellamy at Time-Life for help at every step along the way, and to my loving wife and children.

To your good health and good cheer,

Mo Siegel

About the Author

Mo Siegel, a naturalist and entrepreneur, founded Celestial Seasonings at the age of 20. Suffering from asthma as a child, Mo committed himself to discovering and sharing the natural secrets of good health. That search led directly to hand-picking and blending the wondrous herbs growing wild in the Rocky Mountains—which became the first Celestial tea blends. Today, the company serves over 1.5 billion cups of tea a year and is America's largest herb provider. Mo is an avid outdoorsman, father, health advocate, businessman, and connoisseur of good-for-you herbs and teas.

- CONTENTS -

PART I

HERBS FOR HEALTH

Soothing Aches and Pains

Herbal first aid for arthritis; bruises, burns, and cuts; backaches; muscle pain, sprains, and spasms; earaches, headaches, and toothaches

Fighting Colds, Flus, and Allergies

Herbal relief for sneezing, coughing, and congestion; fever, chills, and body aches; sore throat and aching head; itchy and irritated eyes; upset stomach, nausea, and vomiting

Maintaining Healthy Skin

Herbal remedies for acne; athlete's foot and other fungal infection; boils; cold sores; eczema and hives; dry or sunburned skin; poison ivy and poison oak; psoriasis; warts

Building a Healthy Heart

Using herbs to help strengthen your cardiovascular system, lower cholesterol, manage high blood pressure, and ease the pain of angina

Calming an Upset Stomach

Using herbs to relieve constipation, diarrhea, flatulence and gas, indigestion, irritable bowel, and nausea and vomiting

Embracing Good Reproductive Health

Safe and natural herbs for treating menopause, menstrual problems, osteoporosis, PMS, and the prostate

Strengthening Your Immune System

Using herbs to support, stimulate, and regulate your immune system and to help prevent and treat cancer

C O N T E N T S

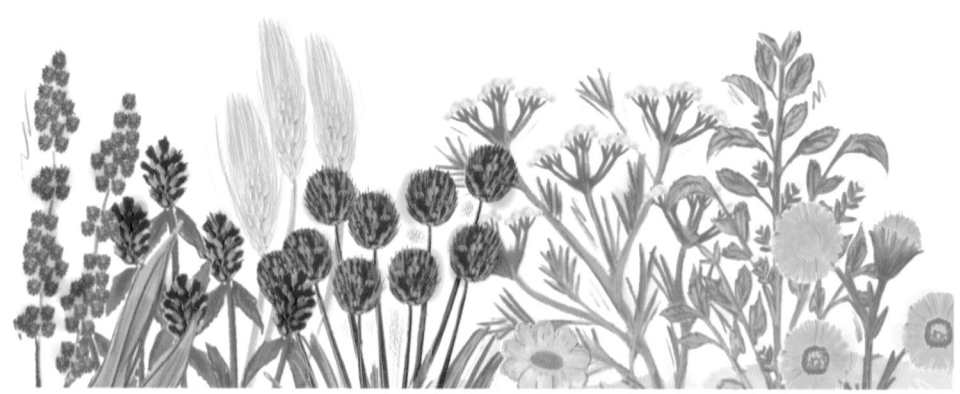

INTRODUCTION

by Mo Siegel

Mountains should be climbed with as little effort as possible and without desire. . . .
If you become restless, speed up. If you become winded, slow down.
You climb the mountain in an equilibrium between restlessness and exhaustion. . .
each footstep isn't just a means to an end, but a unique event in itself.
—ROBERT M. PIRSIG

Mountains and plants are my joy and my inspiration, the symbols of my passion for everything pure, natural, and good for body and soul. Indeed, I cut my teeth—and found my true heart's calling—in the meadows and highlands of the great Rocky Mountains. Palmer Lake, Colorado, where I was raised, is a small mountain town surrounded by nature's sumptuous bounty. My world was (and still is) a place of richly scented pine trees, fields of wild flowers and plants, invigorating clean air, and snow-capped Rockies silhouetted against blue Colorado sky.

As a child, I suffered from severe asthma. While lying in my mountain bed, gasping for enough air to breathe, I made a lifetime commitment to fight my way to good health. And somewhere along the journey, that commitment grew into a passion for bringing great tasting and healthy herbs to the public.

By the summer of my nineteenth year, I was intoxicated with the wonders of the natural world and an avid hiker, mountain climber, and health food fanatic. That summer, during hikes in the highlands around the Rockies, I discovered the abundance of wild and healthful herbs growing there. Like many of my contemporaries in the '60s and '70s, I had become a passionate advocate of natural, healthful foods, as well as a lover of soothing herbal teas—most of which were either imported or hard to find and buy in the States. The wild herbs I discovered that summer started me thinking about making my own herbal brews. I would pick herbs, blend them into teas, and serve the teas to my friends. Thanks to their encouragement, I hatched a plan to gather healthy herbs in the wild and make them into the finest tasting teas available in the United States.

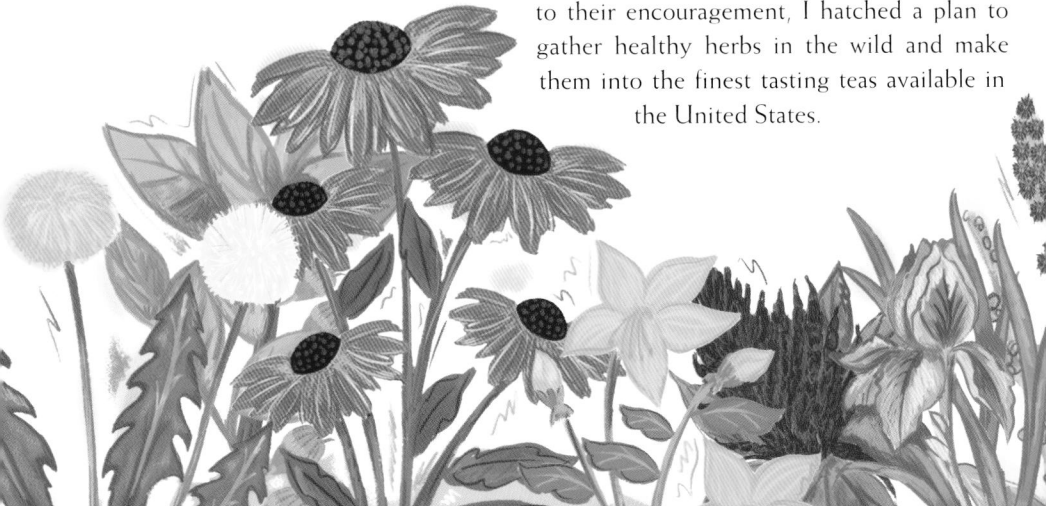

During the next winter, I learned everything I could about combining healthful herbs into delicious teas. By the following summer, several close friends and I started hiking the mountain meadows and harvesting wild herbs. Raspberry and red clover, chamomile and peppermint, were some of the many plants we first gathered. We dried the leaves, buds, and flowers on old screen doors set out in the Colorado sun. By the end of the summer, we had harvested, cured, and blended 36 different herbs—what became MO'S 36 HERB TEA, our first natural herb product and the genesis of Celestial Seasonings.

Over 25 years and thousands of tea blends later—soothing teas, invigorating teas, delicious teas, exotic teas, and healing teas; teas that feature more than 100 herbs, fruits, and spices from around the world—Celestial Seasonings is going stronger than ever. In recent years, as people increasingly needed alternative ways to maintain good health and fight illness, we naturally expanded our world of beverage teas to include healing herbal formulas and herbal medicines, supplemented with vitamins and nutrients.

While the natural products we offer have grown in number, and our harvesting and manufacturing methods have changed, our fundamental aims and beliefs haven't. And never will. We aim to celebrate life and good health by giving you the best of what is pure, natural, and healthful—whether it be teas or herbal supplements. And we aim to deliver good health in the same way we make our herbal products, with commitment, love, passion, and a dash of whimsy—just like the quotations featured on our packaging and in this book.

What we believe in is the extraordinary power of plants, particularly medicinal plants. We believe in the power of leaves, roots, blossoms, and seeds—made into teas, capsules, tinctures, or oils—to restore and maintain good health, to nourish and sustain the body, to calm and strengthen the mind, to soothe and uplift the soul.

This book celebrates the power of healing plants and the role they play in supporting health and happiness. Herbs aren't panaceas, of course, nor simple means to an end. Health and happiness are sometimes elusive and hard-won goals—like a cloud-covered mountain peak when you are only halfway up the slope and already tired and hungry. But herbs can provide potent support and healing along the way to good health and a happy heart. Enjoy the journey.

Mo Siegel
BOULDER, COLORADO
JULY 1999

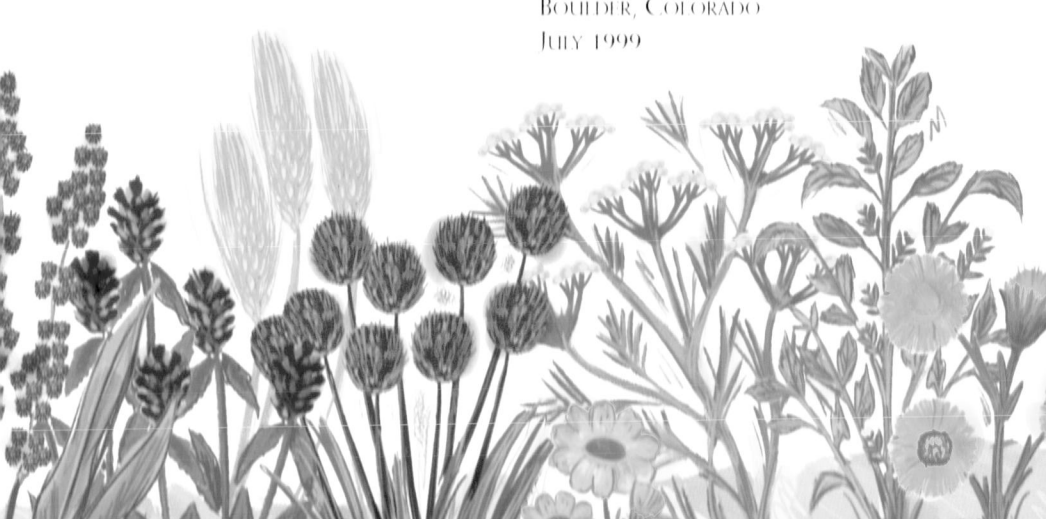

THE WHYS AND HOWS OF USING THIS BOOK

Our love affair with plants—with both the beauty and the healing they provide body and soul—can be traced back to a time before written history, some even say as far back as Neanderthal man, but certainly to at least 10,000 years ago. It was then, about 8,000 B.C., that Neolithic humans (as archaeologists have proven) gathered around their home fires not only the first tools for farming, but also the leaves, roots, and seeds of medicinal and household plants such as vervain, elderberry, fumitory, and soapwort. Amazingly, we still use the same plant herbs today. Indeed, all four are featured in this book.

Perhaps it was in the New Stone Age, then, among the misty lakeside dwellings of Neolithic man and woman, that herbal medicine was truly born. And along with that birthing came the first attempts to record for posterity the mysteries of plant medicine. What we would later call "herbals" and "pharmacopoeias" and "materia medica"—all names for formal written records identifying herbs and how to use them—began many millennia ago as oral teachings passed down from generation to generation. When humans began to write, they roughly carved their herbal knowledge into shells and stones. Later, they took to ink and inscribed sheets of papyrus and parchment with the wonders of healing plants.

This well of herbal knowledge grew deeper and richer in the centuries that followed: from the golden herbal ages of Egypt, Greece, Rome, India, and China, to the herbal theories of Anglo-Saxon alchemists in the Middle Ages; from the classic seventeenth-century British herbals of John Gerard and Nicholas Culpeper, to the earthy synthesis of Old European and Native American herb lore in Colonial America; from the late twentieth-century demand for natural and inexpensive alternative medicines, to modern science's headline-grabbing testaments to the value of many, many herbs. Now comes this latest homage to herbal medicine, which you hold in your hands—*Herbs for Health & Happiness.*

Another herbal? Yes, but one with a twist. You'll find no A-to-Z listing of herbs here (except for a short guide in the appendix), nor even an alphabetical listing of ailments. Here we don't treat health and herbs as static entities that have narrowly defined causes and effects. Herbal medicine is holistic and synergistic. It treats the whole person and the interplay of body, mind, and soul in fostering health and happiness. Herbs themselves are holistic entities. Unlike conventional drugs, herbs have multiple healing actions that balance and support each other and are the result of intricate interactions between hundreds of plant chemicals. One specific herb may treat several different ailments. Several complementary herbs combined may be the most effective treatment for one distinct malady.

Our book celebrates these holistic dimensions of herbal medicine. Here we look at herbs in the most basic of ways: how they can help people find those passionately sought-after goals—good health and simple happiness. And we not only provide you with the herbal know-how for restoring and maintaining health and happiness, we also sprinkle the book with helpful tips on everything from making herbal baths and hot toddies, to using yoga to relieve indigestion. And we add a goodly dash of optimism and humor to this healthful brew by weaving inspiring quotations throughout the book's pages—because sometimes, all you need to jump-start health and happiness is a jolt of simple hope and good cheer.

In the first half of the book, we focus on good health and offer herbal remedies for relieving pain, fighting colds and allergies, treating skin ailments, healing the heart, calming upset stomachs, nourishing the reproductive organs, and strengthening immunity. If you've been avoiding dinner parties because indigestion and gas is the bane of your existence, open up to "Calming an Upset Stomach," and you'll find a wide selection of herbs that gently heal the tummy.

In the second part of the book, where the focus is happiness, we recommend herbs for soothing anxiety and stress, boosting energy, relieving insomnia, and treating depression, as well as herbal help for losing weight and practicing natural beauty. If you've begun forgetting where you put your car keys or your reading glasses (or your ten-year-old Toyota on trips to the mall), turn to the pages of "Sharpening Your Memory" for herbal hints on how to maximize brain power.

Each herb discussed is accompanied by its common English and Latin names, a short history, some whimsical legends and lore about the herb, the most common ailments for which the herb is prescribed and why, and the most common forms in which the herb can be bought. And if one herb is good for treating several health conditions, you'll see the herb reappear in slightly different forms in other chapters. Along the way, you'll also find cautions, warnings, and special notes about specific herbs and health conditions—we urge you to read them.

A special note: We almost never recommend doses in this book. That's because we encourage you to work with a qualified practitioner. Herbs are medicine. Some must be taken with care, and others should be avoided. An herbal practitioner can help you make the right choices for your needs. Of course, many herbs are so safe that you can find them commercially made and readily available in herb markets, health food stores, Asian pharmacies, supermarkets, and drug store chains. We encourage you to try the best of these commercial herbal medicines, but again—and especially if you take other medications or have a chronic illness—only after talking with your practitioner.

Mostly, we welcome you to the wonderful world of herbal medicine and hope you'll bring an open heart and sense of adventure to the joyous task of embracing health and happiness for the journey through life—whatever your life and that journey may be. Trust, as we do, that the herbs offered here will provide incomparable support, strength, nourishment, and healing along the way.

How to Take Your Herbal Medicine

Although we don't offer dosage information in this book, most of the herbs we feature can safely be taken in tea form—perhaps the best and easiest way to get all of an herb's healing benefits. You can find many herbal teas already prepackaged in commercial preparations. But some herbs may only be available in chopped, dried, or fresh herb form. You can easily make your own teas at home, however, and enjoy them when you need them.

To make a healing herbal tea, place 1 tablespoon of dried herb or 2 tablespoons of fresh herb in a tea pot or cup with lid. Pour 8 ounces of boiling spring water over the herb, cover the pot or cup, and steep for 10 to 15 minutes. Strain and add honey, if you like. If you are making a tea out of the harder parts of a plant, such as the roots, rhizomes, or seeds, place the same amount of ingredients given above directly into the boiling water, cover the pot, simmer for 15 to 20 minutes, then strain. Tea made this way is called a decoction.

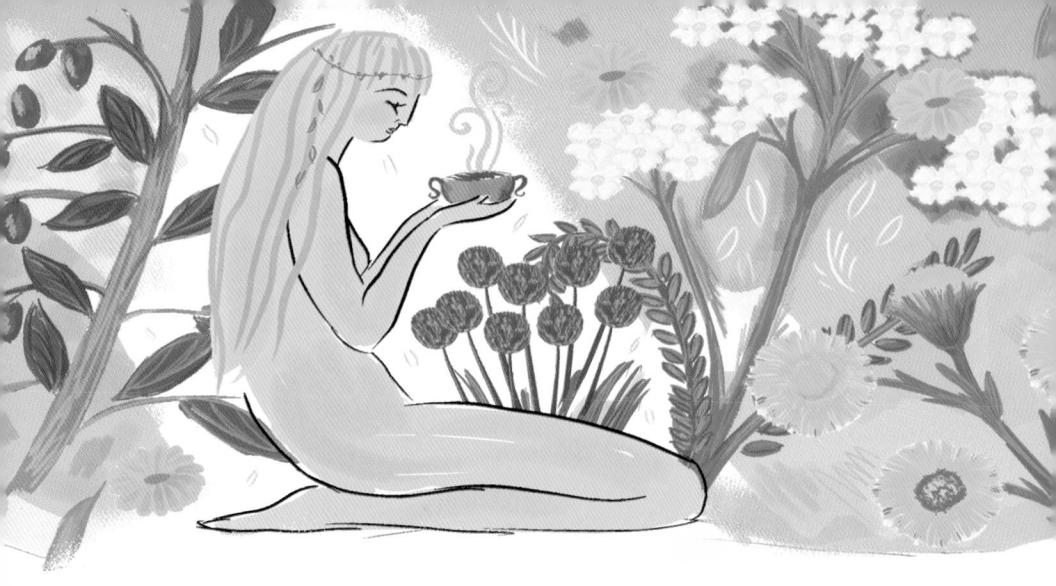

herbs
for
HEALTH

Nicholas Culpeper, the renowned seventeenth-century herbalist, probably did more for mainstream herbal medicine than did any other herbalist of his time or later. Most notably, he translated Britain's official—and sacrosanct—herbal pharmacopoeia from Latin to English and thus made herbal medicine available to the working class for the first time. That translation became the famed *Culpeper's Complete Herbal*, and it is still in use today.

But Culpeper wasn't perfect, and he certainly wasn't always right. For one thing, he believed the planets and stars ruled the properties of

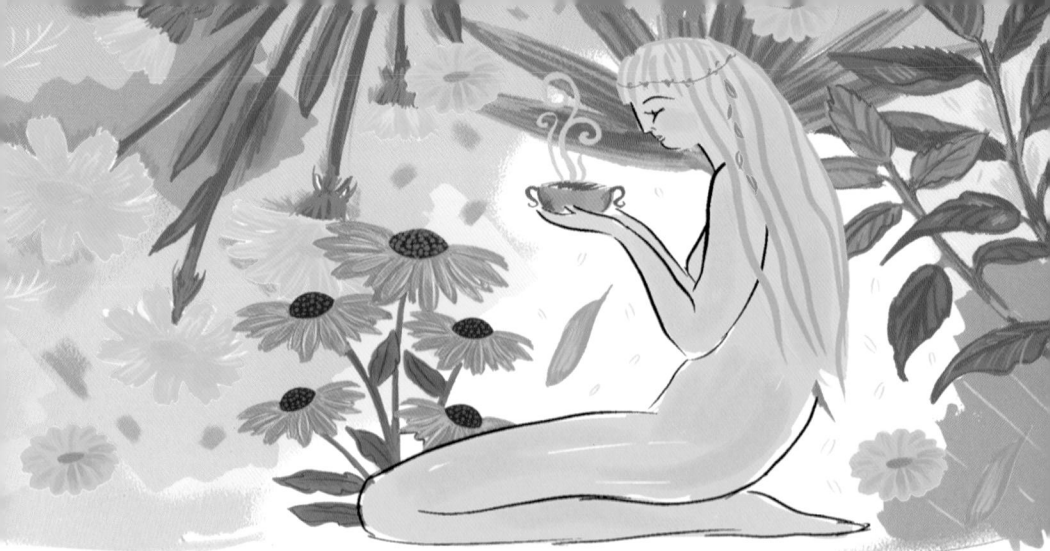

herbs. Motherwort, for example, was ruled by sensual Venus and thus could "settle the womb" and cure "the trembling of the heart." As unscientific as that sounds, today motherwort is indeed used to regulate menstruation and ease heart palpitations.

Yet when it came to garlic (ruled by fiery Mars), Culpeper was sharply off the mark. He hated the stuff and believed it did as much harm as good: ". . . let it be taken inwardly with great moderation; outwardly you may make more bold with it."

Today, of course, many people "make bold" with garlic and would never consider taking it in "moderation." Instead, it is an integral part of many heart-healthy diets.

Nevertheless, we open with this cautionary fable by way of warning you to take your herbal medicine with a grain of common sense. Herbs are a wonderful and mostly safe way to treat many ailments. But herbs are drugs, albeit natural ones, and like conventional drugs, they should be used responsibly and moderately. Herbs are not cure-alls. The same herb that works for one person may not work for another. Some herbs (and conventional drugs) work well together. Other herbs don't mix well at all—with anything. If you are new to using herbs or have a pre-existing health problem, talking to a qualified medical practitioner is a must.

Other than that proviso, enjoy discovering the healing power of herbs. And take all the garlic you want. Your heart will love you for it.

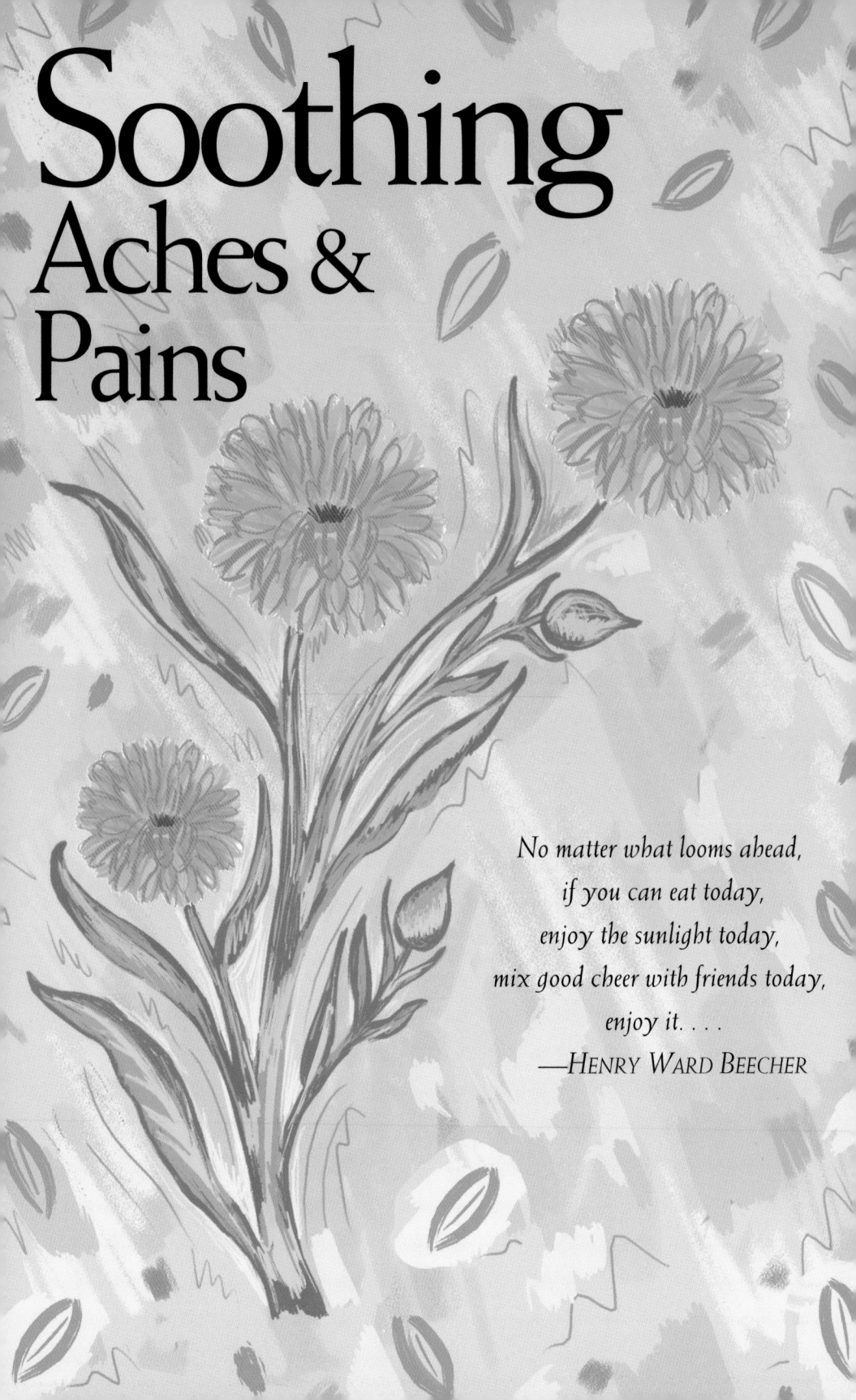

Soothing
Aches &
Pains

No matter what looms ahead,
if you can eat today,
enjoy the sunlight today,
mix good cheer with friends today,
enjoy it. . . .
—HENRY WARD BEECHER

PAIN

No one person's pain is like another's. Whether chronic or acute, dull or sharp, pain—how we perceive it, endure it, and treat it—is a unique and personal phenomenon. The acute cramping pain that incapacitates one individual may be nothing more than a chronic nuisance to another.

In fact, many of us strike an uneasy peace with chronic pain almost every day. We learn to live with arthritic and rheumatic pain in the body's joints and connective tissues; with stress- and injury-related muscle pains and spasms; with the nagging tension headaches and ubiquitous lower back pain that seem emblematic of our late-millennial lifestyles.

Still others of us—probably most of us—can barely tolerate the short-lived but acutely painful occurrences of earaches, toothaches, cuts, bruises, and burns that are often part of daily life.

Like it or not, pain is essential to our ultimate wellness. It is a physiological red flag, the nervous system's way of alerting us that some part of the body is injured, infected, or diseased. Pain is usually the first warning we have that something has gone wrong with our bodies. Consequently, any frontline defense against pain first begins with a look at its underlying cause, particularly if the pain is accompanied by serious injury, fever, inflammation, or nausea, or if the pain is new, sudden, acute, or debilitating. A consultation with your medical practitioner is a must.

But once an underlying problem is either ruled out or identified and treated, many herbs can effectively and naturally relieve pain—and even more. Because almost all herbs have several synergistic therapeutic properties, the greatest pain-relieving (or analgesic) herbs will often also target the underlying causes of pain: infection, inflammation, fever, muscular spasms, and cramps. The following are some of the finest pain-relieving herbs that the plant kingdom has to offer. Most of them also have antibacterial, anti-inflammatory, fever-reducing, and anti-spasmodic properties.

*[Nature] is the one place
where miracles not only happen,
but happen all the time.
—THOMAS WOLFE*

GENERAL ACHES AND PAINS

ARNICA
(Arnica montana)

Among all the pain-relieving and wound-healing herbs, the yellow-flowered arnica plant reigned supreme among folk herbalists for centuries. Also known as sneezewort and leopard's bane, extracts of arnica's daisy-like flowers are today used in oils, creams, ointments, teas, and compresses to relieve pain—especially the acute pain of sudden injuries—and to hasten healing for a variety of ailments. These include bruises, sprains, sports injuries, muscle and joint pain, and slow-to-heal wounds and bone fractures. Applied externally in a compress, arnica is especially beneficial in relieving the painful swelling of arthritis and rheumatism.

The dried herb or tincture (called *Arnica tinctura*) is available in pharmacies and health food stores. Arnica is also available in commercially prepared ointments and creams. Follow your practitioner's or the manufacturer's directions.

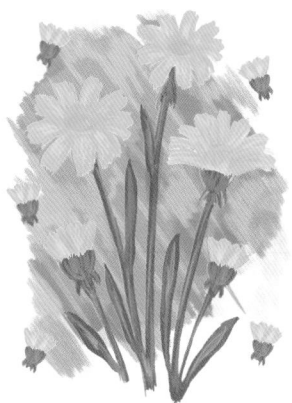

ARNICA
(Arnica montana)

Caution: Arnica is extremely toxic when taken internally. Since 1968 it has been approved only for external use. Keep herbal solution away from children and animals, and discard leftover herb and used compresses immediately.

CHAMOMILE
(Matricaria chamomilla [German], Anthemis nobilis [Roman])

Generally celebrated as a tea that calms, sedates, and promotes sleep, the essential oils of the chamomile plant also have analgesic, antispasmodic, and antiseptic properties. Thus herbalists have long used chamomile to treat pain, muscular spasms, and infections—as well as stress and anxiety. In Germany, chamomile's many therapeutic uses have earned it the nickname *alles zutraut* ("can do anything"), and ancient Egyptians believed it could even slow the aging process. Variously called whig plant, ground apple, and *manzanilla* ("little apple"), the crushed flowers of the chamomile plant have a sweet, apple-like taste and odor and can be eaten on their own or in salads.

More commonly, chamomile is taken internally as a tea—three or four cups a day— to relieve muscular cramping and pain. It may also be used as an inhalant to relieve the pain and congestive swelling of sinusitis. Applied externally, chamomile compresses can reduce the swelling and ease the pain of arthritic joints and stiff muscles and speed the healing of burns and wounds. Chamomile is widely available in commercial preparations of dried herb, tincture, or tea. Follow the manufacturer's directions.

WHITE WILLOW
(Salix alba)

According to esteemed seventeenth-century British herbalist and astrologer Nicholas

Culpeper, to whom we owe much of our seminal knowledge about Western herbs, both the willow and the wintergreen trees (discussed later) are ruled by the cold and arid moon. This apparently accounted for the "cooling" and "drying" properties that traditionally made both herbs such fine vulneraries (wound healers). Indeed, willow was historically used primarily to stanch bleeding.

Modern science, however, identified willow just over 100 years ago as a member of the potent salicin-producing plant family—the salicylates—that are superior pain relievers and fever reducers. Salicin became the precursor of the most celebrated drug in pharmaceutical history, aspirin.

Willow is in demand again today as a "natural" aspirin that relieves many aches and pains with far less stomach irritation than aspirin. The bark of the willow tree is most potent and is available as tea, dried herb, tincture, and capsules. Follow the manufacturer's directions.

Caution: Do not use white willow with other salicylates, such as aspirin or wintergreen, because of the danger of heightened side effects such as severe stomach upset and nausea. Do not give to children with colds because of the risk of Reye's syndrome. Adults with stomach disorders should not use White Willow.

WINTERGREEN
(Gaultheria procumbens)

Gaultherin, one of the primary chemical constituents in the wintergreen plant, is similar in structure to the salicylates in "natural" aspirin-like herbs such as willow and meadowsweet. Like those plants, wintergreen is an effective general pain reliever and anti-inflammatory that may be particularly useful in treating the pain of arthritis, rheumatism, and musculoskeletal ailments such as sprains, spasms, and joint and tissue injuries.

Also called teaberry, mountain tea, and checkerberry, the leaves of the wintergreen plant are made into an aromatic tea. Wintergreen oil is also available in creams and salves and can be applied directly to painful joints and muscles.

Caution: Follow the same precautions as indicated for white willow.

Work That Body!

Don't just sit there—put down the book and do something! Take a brisk walk around the neighborhood. Rake the leaves. Bike down to the convenience store. Mop the kitchen floor. Challenge your kids to a race. Take the dog for a run.

Besides helping to strengthen the heart and lose weight, moderate exercise has benefits that are especially good for those who suffer chronic pain or joint ailments such as arthritis. Consider some of these exercise bonuses:

- Strengthens bones and muscles
- Increases flexibility
- Releases pain-relieving, feel-good endorphins
- Retards aging
- Increases the body's tolerance for stress and pain

To everything there is a season,
and a time to every purpose
under the heaven . . .
A time to weep,
and a time to laugh,
A time to mourn,
and a time to dance.
—*ECCLESIASTES 3:1-8*

ARTHRITIS AND OTHER INFLAMMATORY JOINT AILMENTS

Arthritis refers to inflammation of the joints. The most common form of arthritis is osteoarthritis, which is also known as degenerative joint disease because it is characterized by joint degeneration and loss of cartilage, the shock-absorbing gel-like material between joints. The potential for this degeneration increases as people age.

Rheumatoid arthritis, another common form of arthritis, is an inflammation in the lining of the joints. It can cause damage to cartilage, bone, tendons, ligaments, and other organs. It is considered one of the many chronic, painful, and difficult-to-treat autoimmune disorders. Characteristic traits of rheumatoid arthritis are joints that appear red, spongy, and warm. In osteoarthritis, joints may be cooler and bony hard.

Therapeutic approaches to treating arthritis, rheumatoid arthritis, and other connective tissue and joint ailments often are two-pronged: The first method is symptomatic topical and internal treatment of pain and inflammation with external rubs made with capsaicin (cayenne); the second—particularly in rheumatic ailments—is systemic treatment of suspected underlying infections and toxicity. All the antioxidant herbs, such as Rosemary, are also good systemic treatments for underlying toxicity. Diuretics are often used to eliminate excess fluids and acids. Herbs with antibacterial properties, such as marigold, might also be indicated. In addition to the general pain-relieving herbs already recommended, the following herbs are especially useful in treating arthritis and other painful connective tissue and joint ailments.

BIRCH
(*Betula species*)

Immortalized by the poet Samuel Coleridge as the "Lady of the Woods," the birch tree—also known as cherry birch and sweet birch—has been celebrated throughout history as a symbol of spring and new beginnings. Among the many myths surrounding this ancient tree was the belief that flogging oneself with a birch branch before sunrise on Easter morning would ensure good health for the rest of the year.

The birch's powerfully aromatic leaves, sap, twigs, and bark are similar in taste and smell to wintergreen (*Gaultheria procumbens*) and share some of that plant's healing properties. Rich in essential oils, saponins, and flavonoids, birch is taken internally as a tea made from the bark or leaves. It has excellent anti-inflammatory, pain-relieving, diuretic, and antibacterial properties that are especially effective for treating the symptoms of arthritis, rheumatism, gout, and kidney stones. Birch oil and creams can be applied directly to swollen and painful joints and muscles.

DANDELION
(*Taraxacum officinale*)

One of the most celebrated of medicinal herbs, dandelion has long been used to treat kidney, liver, and gall bladder ailments. Popularly called swine's snout, lion's tooth, and wet-a-bed, among other names, dandelion is one of the best of the herbal diuretics, with the additional advantage of helping the body retain the essential nutrient potassium. Most diuretics leech potassium from the system; dandelion adds potassium. The herb is also a potent antioxidant, rich in vitamins A and C.

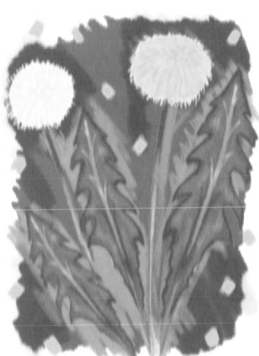

DANDELION
(*Taraxacum officinale*)

Early herbalists believed that dandelion not only helped the body release excess fluids, but was also a general detoxifier, cleansing the body of poisonous substances and excess acids. It is the latter property—as well as dandelion's proven anti-inflammatory action—that makes this herb an excellent treatment for some forms of rheumatism and rheumatic joint ailments. Both conditions are believed to be linked to underlying inflammatory infections and buildups of uric acid.

Both the leaves and roots of the dandelion plant have therapeutic properties, and they are available as tinctures, prepared teas, capsules, and dried herb.

FLAX
(*Linum usitatissimum*)

Also known as flax seed, linseed, and Mary's linen cloth, flax was traditionally used as a laxative and to treat coughs, lung and chest illnesses, and digestive and urinary complaints—uses for which it is still effective today. References to flax's healing properties are found in ancient writings as early as 500 B.C., and as a commercial preparation it appears in Egyptian literature of the fourteenth century B.C. In the Middle Ages, flax flowers were even used to ward off witches!

Therapeutically, flax has a strong demulcent (soothing and moistening) action that heals inflamed membranes and tissues throughout the body. Recent pharmacological research also confirms that flax may be an effective systemic (wide-ranging) treatment for many inflammatory types of arthritis and connective tissue disease because it is rich in health-promoting omega-3 and omega-6 fatty acids (the "good" fats that also lower blood cholesterol). These good fatty acids have been proven to suppress white blood cell production of leukotrienes, fat-like blood particles that cause both arthritic inflammation and some allergic reactions.

The oil extracted from flax seeds can be used both internally (in medications for coughs, colds, sore throats, and general inflammations) and externally (as a therapeutic rub or in warm compresses for painful, inflamed joints and muscles). The crushed seeds can also be wrapped in warm compresses, but they are more popularly used to make a soothing, healing tea.

Caution: Never use commercial linseed oil medicinally.

BRUISES, BURNS, AND CUTS

Bruises The characteristic black-and-blue marks of common bruises are caused by broken, leaking blood vessels beneath injured skin. Cold compresses reduce the pain and swelling of bruises. So too do many plant herbs, but herbs have the added advantages of helping to heal and strengthen injured blood vessels and helping to repair damaged skin tissue.

Burns First-degree burns—the most common type of burn injury—are characterized by painful, reddened skin. A cold compress will help relieve the initial pain, and a variety of soothing herbs can further reduce pain, enhance healing, and fight infection. (Second- and third-degree burns that break the skin and cause blistering should be seen by a medical practitioner.)

Cuts Many common cuts and wounds respond well to herbal treatment. Vul-

nerary herbs help stop bleeding, prevent infection, and reduce inflammation.

The following are some of the best of the pain-relieving and wound-healing herbs for treating minor bruises, burns, and cuts.

*Those who dwell,
as scientists or laymen,
among the beauties and
mysteries of the earth,
are never alone or weary of life. . . .
Those who contemplate
the beauty of the earth
find reserves of strength
that endure as long as life lasts.*
—RACHEL CARSON,
THE SENSE OF WONDER

ALOE
(Aloe vera)

The translucent gel obtained from the inner leaves of this tropical herb, rich in the emollient and soothing polysaccharides, works externally to relieve minor burns, skin irritations, and infections. (Taken internally, aloe also provides relief from stomach disorders.) Among its other ingredients are several that also reduce inflammation. Available in gels and creams, aloe may be applied externally to minor burns, infected wounds, bruises, irritated and painful skin, sunburns, and cuts. Aloe is also available as a powder,

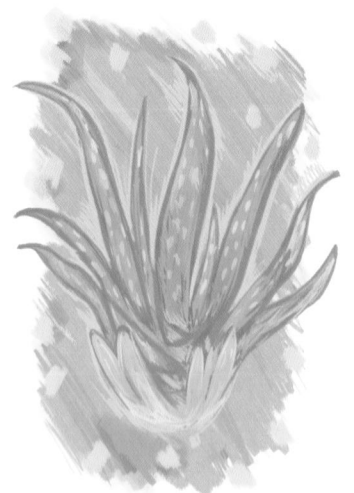

A L O E
(Aloe vera)

a fluid extract, and powdered capsules (for internal use). A soothing mixture combining aloe oil, wheat germ oil, and safflower oil can be applied to bruises to hasten healing and reduce swelling.

MARIGOLD/ CALENDULA
(Calendula officinalis)

The bright orange flowers of the marigold plant are rich with powerful antiseptic (antibacterial), anti-inflammatory, antispasmodic, and wound-healing properties, making marigold—or calendula as it is sometimes more popularly known—one of the finest herbs for treating wounds, skin abrasions, and infections. (Taken internally it also alleviates indigestion.)

Also known as pot marigold, marybud, and holygold, the marigold flower appears frequently in European myths. Young French girls who danced atop a bed of marigold flowers were believed to be able to talk with birds. A gypsy legend has it that a potion of marigold flowers allowed one to see the fairies.

High in the antioxidant vitamin C, and bitterly astringent, marigold is excellent for stopping bleeding and hastening the closing of slow-to-heal wounds. Available as dried herb or in oils, lotions, creams, and tinctures, marigold can reduce pain and inflammation, prevent infection, and speed healing. Apply it directly to cuts, wounds, sores, burns, and injuries. The leaves of the plant may be mashed and applied directly to burns, and a mixture of goldenseal, calendula, and myrrh makes a fine antiseptic lotion for external use. For a more systemic treatment, drink marigold tea to help reduce the pain and swelling that accompany bruises, burns, and cuts.

BACKACHES

Back pain, especially lower back pain, may seem endemic to our high-tech and unfortunately sedentary lifestyles. Sitting for long periods of time is indeed the worst thing we can do for our backs, and we all do it! In truth, however, backaches have plagued humankind since the beginning of time, and a wide variety of folk remedies to relieve aching backs abound. Good posture, frequent breaks from our desks to stretch and move around, massage, and heat are all tried-and-true, natural treatments. There are also excellent herbal remedies for backache, both to relieve pain and relax muscles.

CRAMP BARK
(Viburnum opulus)

The extraordinary benefits of cramp bark are discussed more extensively in the chapter on optimal reproductive health, where it is featured as the best herb for treating menstrual cramps. It is also an excellent treatment for chronic back pain, particularly lower back pain. The primary healing constituents found in cramp bark (also called Virburnum, European cranberry, and squaw bush) are viburnin, a powerful antispasmodic, and valerianic acid, the same potent sedative found in the herbs valerian and hops. Cramp bark is also an effective anti-inflammatory. Taken internally, cramp bark relaxes muscles, reduces pain and swelling, and exerts a gentle sedating effect. It may also ease the pain of migraines and colic.

The bark of this small tree with tiny white flowers contains the most medicinal properties of the tree and is commonly made into an alcohol-based tincture. Capsules are also available. Follow your practitioner's or the manufacturer's advice.

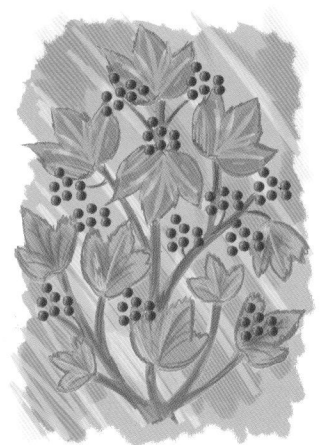

CRAMP BARK
(Viburnum opulus)

The strongest of all warriors are these two—Time and Patience.
—LEO TOLSTOY

YARROW
(Achillea millefolium)

A naturalized perennial from Eurasia, yarrow is widely planted in flower and herb gardens. The herb grows wild in most areas of the United States. In ancient times, yarrow was most frequently used to heal wounds; its other popular names were nosebleed and thousand seal.

Modern science, however, has demonstrated that besides its astringent and antiseptic properties (both of which make it a good wound healer), yarrow also is an effective pain reliever, anti-inflammatory, and mild sedative. The leaves, stems, and flower tops contain more than 10 active ingredients, including salicylic acid (the same ingredient found in white willow and aspirin), menthol, and camphor. Two major chemical constituents, achilletin and achilleine, are thought to help blood coagulate, and thujone (also found in chamomile) has mild sedative properties.

Take internally as a tea to relieve backache, muscular pain, and spasms. Yarrow is available as a prepared tea and as dried herb. Adding honey or molasses relieves the somewhat bitter taste of yarrow tea.

Caution: If you are allergic to ragweed, you may be allergic to yarrow. Do not take yarrow with aspirin or with other herbs containing salicylic acid, such as white willow. Do not give to children.

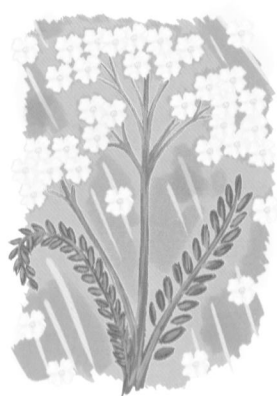

YARROW
(Achillea millefolium)

MUSCLE PAIN, SPRAINS, AND SPASMS

Myalgia is the general term used to describe the constellation of pain, cramping, stiffness, heat, and tenderness that are the hallmark symptoms of a damaged musculoskeletal system—the underlying cause of most acute or chronic muscle pain, sprains, and spasms. Whether the damage is disease-related, as in the case of arthritis, rheumatism, fibromyalgia, and lupus, to name but a few conditions, or the result of sports injuries or accidents, long-standing muscle pain, sprains, and spasms are physically and mentally debilitating. Many herbs provide excellent pain relief for sore and cramped muscles and can reduce inflammation and spasms while targeting any underlying infections or weaknesses in the musculoskeletal system. Here are two of the best.

HYSSOP
(Hyssopus officinalis)

Hyssop, also called sacred herb or holy herb—a reference to its ancient use in cleaning holy places—is a member of the bitter and aromatic mint family. Throughout herbal history it has been used primarily as an expectorant for coughs and other chest complaints. Recent studies of the plant's constituents, however, reveal that hyssop is also a muscle relaxant and gentle sedative. Indeed, taking a hyssop bath or drinking hyssop tea was an old folk remedy for easing the pain of rheumatism.

Hyssop is available as dried or fresh herb—the leaves, flowers, and shoots are often eaten in salads—and as a tincture. To ease muscle pain and spasms, drink hyssop tea or use it in a compress applied directly to sore muscles. A compress may also be used for bruises, burns, and black eyes.

Caution: Hyssop may cause stomach upset and diarrhea.

Life is eternal; and love is immortal; and death is only a horizon; and a horizon is nothing save the limit of our sight.
—ROSSITER WORTHINGTON RAYMOND

VALERIAN
(Valeriana officinalis)

Valerian root, also called vandal root and all-heal, has been used for more than 1,000 years for its calming qualities, and recent research has confirmed its efficacy and safety as a mild tranquilizer and sleep aid.

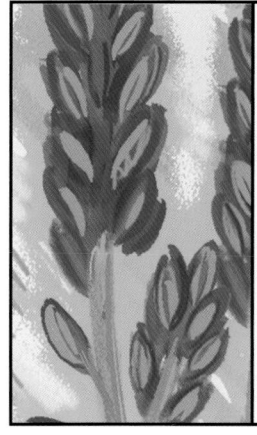

Valerian is also a mild sedative and a superb muscle relaxant, and it can be used to ease the pain and discomfort of muscle cramps, sprains, and spasms. It may also be helpful in relieving the pain of migraines. Two of its main chemical constituents, valerianic and isovalerianic acid, are responsible for valerian's sedating and antispasmodic action. However, unlike its pharmaceutical cousin, Valium, valerian is not habit forming and produces no withdrawal symptoms when discontinued.

It is available in prepared teas—usually in combination with other "calming" herbs—and as dried herb, tinctures, or capsules. Follow the manufacturer's directions on commercial preparations.

Caution: Do not take valerian with conventional tranquilizers or sedatives because of possible enhanced effects.

EARACHES, TOOTHACHES, AND HEADACHES

Earaches Ear infections, especially those accompanied by fever, should be examined by a medical practitioner. Many herbs can also effectively treat ear pain and infection; for example, garlic, in clove or oil form, is a time-honored earache treatment. Here we feature another of the best earache remedies—mullein.

Toothaches Sudden tooth pain is often excruciating and frequently a harbinger of infection. A visit to your dentist is called for if tooth pain lasts for more than a day. In the interim, clove can provide both pain-relieving and infection-fighting properties, as detailed later.

Headaches Headaches come in a variety of forms—in clusters or as migraines; and related to tension, stress, or infection—and they can be as complicated to treat as they are varied in pain and presentation. Here we present three of the best healing herbs for headache pain—cayenne, feverfew, and thyme.

CAYENNE
(Capsicum annuum, C. frutescen, C. minimum)

Cluster headaches differ from tension headaches in that they seem to come in clusters over several hours and are heralded by a mild aching on one side of the head. As the pain becomes more severe, it is usually localized around one eye and accompanied by nasal congestion and flushing. Sinus headaches also are accompanied by nasal congestion, but they are also marked by pain in the forehead and both eyes.

Cayenne and its primary chemical constituent, capsaicin, are wonderfully warming, healing agents long used topically in the treatment of arthritis and other joint ailments. Capsaicin is often the only ingredient in many "sports" creams. Applied to the skin, cayenne is warming and relieves muscle and blood vessel spasms. To relieve the pain and accompanying congestion of cluster and sinus headaches, cayenne cream or oil can be placed inside the nostrils and along the bridge of the nose. Rubbing some cayenne ointment on the temples and along the bridge of the nose may even prevent headaches.

Cayenne or capsaicin creams, ointments, and gels are commercially available. Follow the manufacturer's directions.

Caution: Cayenne is hot! Use sparingly (enough to get an effect) on the skin and inside the nose to avoid burning the skin and membranes.

CLOVE
(*Syzygium aromaticum*)

Clove holds an ancient place in herbalism, having been mentioned in the East by Chinese physicians as early as 400 B.C. and in the West during the time of the Roman scholar Pliny the Elder, who called the aromatic herb caryophyllon (now the name of one of the herb's primary chemical constituents). Rich in stimulating, aromatic essential oils, clove has long been used externally to treat the pain of neuralgia and rheumatism. Internally—usually in combination with other herbs such as chamomile, ginger, linden, or peppermint—it

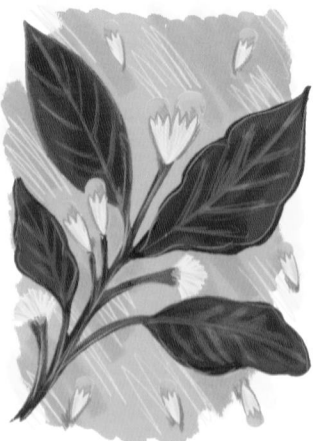

CLOVE
(*Syzygium aromaticum*)

is known to relieve colic, flatulence, nausea, and mild depression.

However, clove is most famed as a remedy for toothache. The dried buds—the same familiar form found in supermarket seasoning sections—can be mashed slightly and held against an aching tooth to temporarily relieve pain. Clove oil is also commercially available and may be rubbed directly on a sore tooth or gum for short periods, or applied to cotton or gauze and then placed on the tooth.

Caution: Prolonged use of cloves or clove oil may seriously irritate gums or damage nerves in the teeth. Consult a medical practitioner for any severe tooth or gum pain that does not resolve in a day.

FEVERFEW
(*Tanacetum parthenium* or *Chrysanthemum parthenium*)

The most frequently recommended herb for treating and preventing the debilitating pain of migraine headaches is feverfew. This daisy-like member of the chrysanthemum family, also known as featherfew and featherfoil, was used historically by folk herbalists to treat fevers, colic, neuralgia, earache, and rheumatism. It was even applied externally in tincture form as an insect repellent. Today, feverfew is most famous for relieving pain when many other conventional and alternative treatments have failed.

The primary chemical constituent in feverfew, the chemical parthenolide, appears to act as a histamine blocker, both reducing histamine production and blocking the release of these inflammatory substances into the blood. These histamines appear to play a key role in the onset of migraine headaches.

Feverfew not only helps reduce the pain of an acute migraine attack, but long-term therapy with feverfew may eventually prevent migraines altogether. Fresh feverfew leaves, chewed daily, are considered the most effective way to get immediate relief from migraine pain and debilitation, but feverfew is also available as dried herb, pills, capsules, and tinctures. Follow your practitioner's or the manufacturer's directions and be patient. It may take two to three months of using feverfew daily to significantly reduce or completely prevent the incidence of migraines.

Caution: Chewing fresh feverfew leaves may cause mouth sores or abdominal pain. If either occur, discontinue using the herb and consult a medical practitioner.

MULLEIN
(Verbascum thapsus)

The long yellow-flowered stalks and oversized leaves of the mullein plant have contributed to the herb's many whimsical popular names, including bunny's ears, donkey's ears, and fatleaf (*gordolobo* in Latin American countries). In folk medicine, where mullein was believed to be a magical herb of the ancient gods, the plant's leaves

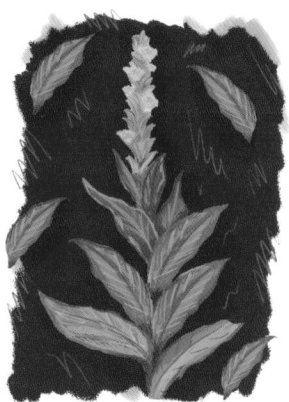

MULLEIN
(Verbascum thapsus)

and flowers were (and sometimes still are) smoked in pipes and handmade cigarettes to relieve asthma and other respiratory problems, including bronchitis.

Mullein flowers also have emollient, antiseptic, and anti-inflammatory properties that make them soothing and healing treatments for common earaches and ear infections. Mullein oil (usually a combination of crushed mullein flowers and olive oil) is available in herb shops and health food stores. Place two or three drops in the outer part of the ear for pain relief and prevention of infection. (Garlic is also used in a similar manner to treat earaches and infection. In fact, a crushed clove may be placed directly in the ear.)

Caution: If earache continues for more than a day or two, especially with fever, or if an underlying infection is suspected, see a medical practitioner immediately.

THYME
(Thymus vulgaris)

It may be one of the most famous culinary herbs worldwide, but for tension headaches, nothing beats a cup of cold thyme tea. (Hot thyme tea, on the other hand, is used to treat insomnia, stomach cramps, whooping cough, and diarrhea, among other ailments.) A dull, persistent, nonthrobbing pain that envelops the whole head and often the neck characterizes tension headaches. They are commonly triggered by stress, and thyme can be a real rescue remedy.

Also known as mother thyme, black thyme, and common thyme, the plant's sharply aromatic essential oils are responsible for most of its therapeutic actions, which are largely antiseptic and antispasmodic. The chemical constituents thymol and carvacrol account for more than half of thyme's essential oils, and both are strong antiseptics that can quickly soothe congested mucous membranes and calm throbbing muscles and nerves.

The dried herb, made from crushed leaves and flower tops, is widely available and may be made into a tea for relieving the pain of tension headaches.

More
Helpful Advice

GOOD-FOR-YOU FOODS, FATS, AND SUGAR!

The right food, vitamins, and supplements can go a long way to alleviating arthritis pain, replacing lost cartilage, and repairing joint damage. Follow these guidelines:

■ Avoid caffeine, dairy products, tomatoes and potatoes (which can aggravate arthritis symptoms) and eat a low-protein, reduced meat diet. Both measures can help relieve arthritis pain and promote collagen production (which is essential to repairing cartilage).

■ Include plenty of the "good fats"—omega-6 and omega-3—in your diet. These essential fatty acids produce natural anti-inflammatories in the body called prostaglandins which reduce inflammation and relieve pain. You can find good fats in grape seed oil, soybeans, salmon, sardines, canola oil, sesame oil, and flax seeds, among other foods.

■ Get at least the minimum daily requirements of vitamin A, which destroys damage-causing free radicals, and vitamins C, B_6, B_3, and E, which promote collagen production and tissue repair.

■ Supplement your diet with glucosamine and chondroitin, special nutrients in the body's tissues that help in the formation of bones and tendons, repair damaged joints, and rebuild cartilage. You can find both supplements in capsule form as glucosamine sulfate and chondroitin sulfate.

Fighting
Colds, Flus, & Allergies

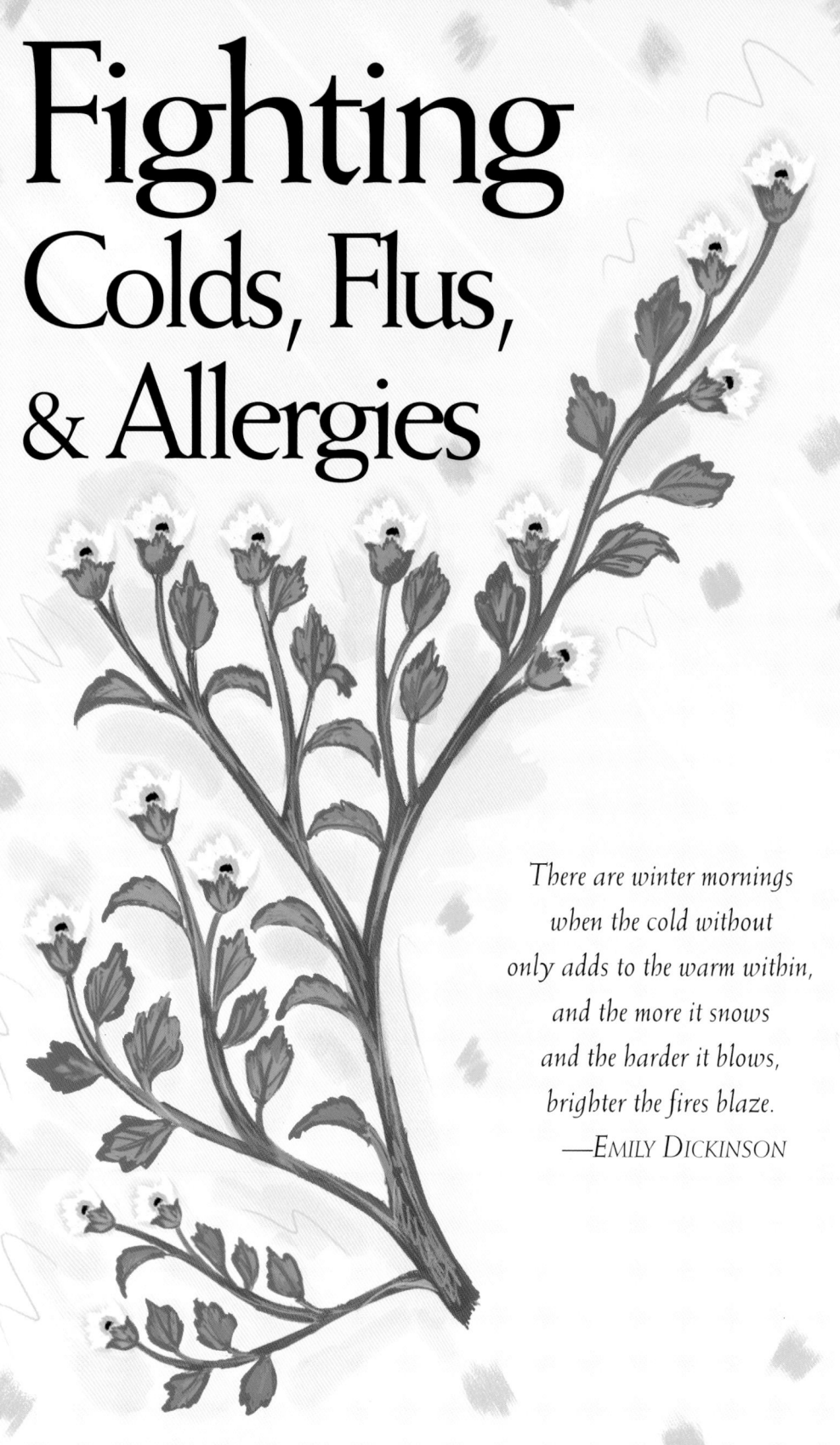

*There are winter mornings
when the cold without
only adds to the warm within,
and the more it snows
and the harder it blows,
brighter the fires blaze.*
—EMILY DICKINSON

COLDS, FLUS, AND ALLERGIES

Colds and Flus The common cold and flu (influenza) are caused by viruses—in fact, by any of several hundred viruses—and there are no cures for these contagious, debilitating, and commonplace viral ailments. Antibiotics—notoriously overprescribed and overused—have their place in medicine, but only against bacterial infections. Against viruses they are useless.

The first line of defense against colds and flus is to maintain a strong and healthy body that supports the immune system's ability to fight off any infection. When cold and flu viruses do attack—heralded by a host of symptoms that can include sneezing, coughing, congestion, fever, chills, body aches, sore throat, irritated eyes, nausea, and vomiting—the second line of defense is fast and safe symptomatic relief. From the moment humankind began self-treating their aches and pains with plants, a variety of herbs have been used safely and successfully to relieve cold and flu symptoms. Some of the best—both for prevention and for symptomatic relief—are presented here.

Allergies Allergies, on the other hand, occur when the immune system overreacts to one or more of a legion of irritants (allergens) that plague allergy sufferers: dust mites, pollen, pollutants, animal dander, fungi, spores, medications, bee stings, and food products. By far the most common of allergies is hay fever, or allergic rhinitis; more than 20 percent of the American population endure cold-like hay fever symptoms each spring when trees are pollinating.

Some allergies can be life threatening and must be managed by conventional medications and interventions. Included among these are allergies to penicillin, bee stings, and certain foods such as peanuts.

Hay fever, however, is not life threatening, although it certainly can be disabling. The immune system reacts to the offending allergen pollen by releasing histamine, a powerful chemical substance that is itself an irritant and causes much of the swelling, congestion, sneezing, coughing, and scratchy throat and eyes that characterize hay fever. In the process of fighting the allergen, histamine can damage delicate tissues and mucous membranes in the eyes, nose, throat, chest, and lungs, which in turn may precipitate secondary infections such as sinusitis.

Conventional allergy drugs (antihistamines) relieve allergy symptoms but often do further damage to tissues and mucus membranes because of their strong "drying" or astringent action. They may also cause drowsiness or heart palpitations, and they do nothing to support or stimulate the immune system.

Many of the same herbs that relieve cold and flu symptoms and bolster the immune system's defenses against infection are also effective in relieving allergy symptoms, soothing the damage to delicate tissues and mucous membranes, and enhancing the body's overall immunity to allergens.

Let's start by looking at those herbs that may prevent or reduce viral infections and common allergies. Later, in Chapter 7 ("Strengthening Your Immune System"), we discuss the immune-stimulating herbs more extensively.

FIGHTING COLDS, FLUS, AND ALLERGIES

ASTRAGALUS
(Astragalus membranaceus)

An immune-bolstering staple of traditional Chinese medicine (TCM) for thousands of years, astragalus (*Huang qi* in TCM) is now the subject of considerable Western research. Asian and Western herbalists—who commonly know the plant as milk vetch root—have long used astragalus to strengthen the body's resistance to infection and to relieve cold and flu symptoms and ailments of the lungs. In the last decade conventional medical science has confirmed the herb's therapeutic properties. Studies have shown that the polysaccharides in astragalus stimulate the immune system, generally strengthen the body overall, promote tissue regeneration, and increase energy. One study demonstrated that astragalus not only reduced the incidence of colds but also shortened the length of cold infection.

The dried powdered root of the plant is available as a prepared tea and in fluid, extract, capsule, and powdered forms. Follow your medical practitioner's or the manufacturer's directions. The herb may also be added to soups and grain dishes and eaten as a daily supplement.

ECHINACEA
(Echinacea purpurea, E. pallida, E. angustifolia)

Popularly known as the purple coneflower, echinacea has long been believed to strengthen the body's defenses against infection. Many Native American tribes regularly used echinacea in poultices, mouthwashes, and teas to heal insect stings, snake bites, and infected wounds; the raw root was chewed to relieve toothaches. Early American herbalists similarly used echinacea to fight infection and relieve cold and flu symptoms. In fact, the United States Dispensatory—a precursor of the U.S. Food and Drug Administration (FDA)—listed echinacea as an infection fighter more than 100 years ago, although the herb fell out of favor after 1910 when it was proclaimed "worthless" by the American Medical Association.

Today echinacea has reemerged as one of the superherbs of the plant kingdom. Practitioners and patients alike prize the dried root worldwide as both an immune stimulant and an infection fighter. Studies have shown that as an infection fighter, echinacea appears to have broad-based antiviral and antibacterial actions against many types of illnesses, including colds, flus, bronchitis, and ear infections. It also

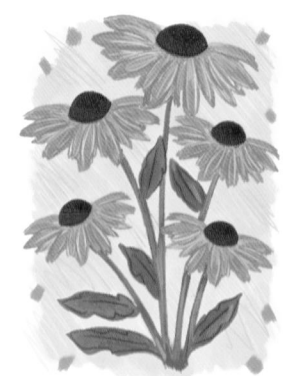

ECHINACEA
(Echinacea purpurea, E. pallida,
E. angustifolia)

seems to stimulate and support the immune system's white blood cells in their battle against viral and bacterial invaders.

Taken internally for colds, flu, and other respiratory illnesses, echinacea is available in tea, capsule, tincture, and dried bulk form. Follow your practitioner's or the manufacturer's direction.

Caution: Do not take echinacea or other immune-boosting herbs if you have any autoimmune disorder.

GARLIC
(Allium sativum)

The seventeenth-century herbalist Nicholas Culpeper reminded us that garlic, a member of the onion family, was considered the "poor man's treacle" in ancient times. Garlic does indeed have an esteemed history among the "working man." Egyptian slaves building the great pyramid of Cheops were fed garlic cloves daily to help keep up their strength.

Garlic is also known as "devil's posy," from the folk belief that when Satan stepped out of Paradise after the Fall, the garlic plant sprung up where his foot landed. Indeed, garlic has a long association

with evil and magic, due no doubt in part to its noxious odor. This is an especially ironic association because garlic has an equally long history in both Chinese and Western herbalism as a broad-spectrum infection fighter and general strengthening tonic for the body.

Allicin, a strong sulphur compound, is the main ingredient of garlic's essential oil and is responsible for its antibiotic, antiseptic, expectorant, and immune-stimulating properties. In China, an extract of allicin is even used in injections to treat various infections. Garlic is also rich in vitamins A, B_1, B_2, and C, and is a superior herb for the cardiovascular system, helping to reduce cholesterol and lower blood pressure (see Chapter 4).

Available as fresh cloves and in tablet form, garlic is taken internally for colds, coughs, and flu. Follow your practitioner's or the manufacturer's directions.

Caution: Garlic contains a chemical that impedes blood clotting. If you have a blood-clotting disorder, consult an herbalist or a healthcare practitioner before using this herb.

NETTLE
(Urtica dioica)

Ancient folk myth has it that rheumatism sufferers would whip their offending joints with the notoriously painful, stinging needles of the nettle plant. The theory behind this self-flagellation was that the pain of the nettle needles would be so bad, it would take the sufferer's mind off his or her rheumatic pain. More likely, the increased blood flow and heat to the rheumatic joint provided the real relief.

Variously known as stinging nettle, Indian spinach, devil's apron, bad-man's-plaything, and hoky-poky, nettle, like garlic, has a long historic connection to things mystical and sometimes nefarious. Scandinavians burned nettles to appease the god Thor and protect their homes from lightning; people of the Middle Ages believed carrying nettle would give them courage and ward off danger and fear.

In truth, nettle—which can be safely used when boiled or dried—has long been used to treat the symptoms of hay fever and to generally reduce an allergic person's sensitivity to allergens, including pollen. The leaves and stems of the nettle plant are rich in vitamins A and C and in calcium, potassium, sulfur, and iron. The herb has both astringent and diuretic properties. The astringent action helps "dry up" and relieve acute allergy symptoms. The diuretic action helps flush chemical toxins from the body and thus supports and strengthens the kidneys and liver.

Taken internally for hay fever symptoms, nettle is available as a tincture, in capsules, and as dried leaves and stems.

Caution: Do not use uncooked nettle; it may cause kidney damage and other symptoms of poisoning.

RELIEVING SYMPTOMS OF COLDS, FLUS, AND ALLERGIES

SNEEZING, COUGHING, AND CONGESTION

Herbs that relieve the sneezing, coughing, and congestion of colds, flus, and allergies generally fall into five types and are often combined in traditional herbal cold and flu formulas. They include:

■ Anti-inflammatories such as coltsfoot, eyebright, marshmallow, mullein, and slippery elm (to treat inflamed and swollen mucous membranes of the nose and throat).

■ Anticatarrhals or antitussives such as coltsfoot and mullein (to stop coughs and relieve congestion and inflammation in the nose and air passages).

■ Astringents such as goldenseal (to help "dry" up a runny nose and clear general congestion).

■ Demulcents such as marshmallow and slippery elm (to soothe irritated and damaged mucous membranes).

■ Expectorants such as coltsfoot and mullein (to break up and stimulate the expulsion [expectoration] of phlegm, especially in the lower respiratory tract).

■ Antispasmodics such as ephedra and black cohosh may also be used if there is difficulty breathing.

The following herbs each have at least one and usually more of these healing properties.

COLTSFOOT
(Tussilago farfara)

Coltsfoot's botanical name derives from the old Latin word tusilago, which means "cough dispeller." The tusilago of ancient Rome became today's antitussives, which are prescribed for coughs and chest congestion.

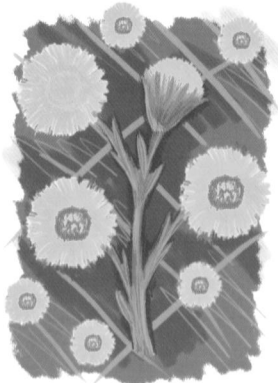

COLTSFOOT
(*Tussilago farfara*)

Also known as coughwort and clatter-cogs, coltsfoot has a renowned place in herbal history as a cough suppressant and gentle expectorant, and it is still used today for those purposes. Coltsfoot also relaxes the bronchial tubes, and nearly 2,000 years ago, the famed Greek botanist Dioscorides recommended that the leaves of coltsfoot be smoked to break up chest congestion. Today, some people still smoke coltsfoot for asthma relief, but increasingly it is taken as a tea or in capsule form under the care of a medical practitioner.

Coltsfoot is prescribed for bronchial congestion, coughs, asthma, and bronchitis. It is available in tincture, capsules, and dried herb (flowers or leaves) form.

A Culinary Note: Coltsfoot pancakes were considered a rare delicacy in the 1700s (the dried leaves were ground and mixed with water to make a batter), and they were often ceremonially served on Shrove Tuesday, the traditional day of merriment and indulgence before Lent begins. Coltsfoot is rich in calcium, potassium, and vitamin C.

Caution: Use coltsfoot only as prescribed by your medical practitioner in moderate to small doses and only for short periods of time. Never give coltsfoot to children, alcoholics, or anyone with liver disease. A small number of studies have reported that coltsfoot can cause liver damage and cancer. Its use is banned in Canada, but not in the United States.

If a man is called
to be a streetsweeper,
he should sweep streets
even as Michelangelo painted,
or Beethoven composed music,
or Shakespeare wrote poetry.
He should sweep streets so well
that all the hosts of heaven
and earth will pause to say,
here lived a great streetsweeper
who did his job well.
—MARTIN LUTHER KING, JR.

MULLEIN
(*Verbascum thapsus*)

A famed herb since medieval times, when the great mystic and amateur botanist Hildegaard of Bingen recommended it for ailments of the chest and lungs, mullein—a member of the snapdragon family—has been used for centuries as an effective expectorant for the coughs and congestion of colds, flus, and bronchitis.

Also known as fluffweed, velvet dock, bunny's ears, and Jacob's staff, mullein's name is a derivation of the Latin word *mollis*, which means "soft," and its velvet-like, soft yellow-gold flowers grow on sturdy stalks that can reach a height of nine feet. In the Middle Ages, the slow-burning stalks were dipped in wax and used as torches.

Almost the whole plant—leaves, flowers, and roots—is rich in mucilage, saponins, and flavonoids, making mullein a gentle expectorant and anti-inflammatory that can soothe and heal swollen mucous membranes. Herbalists prescribe it for a variety of respiratory illnesses with chest and lung complications, and it is often combined with echinacea or elder in cough formulas.

Available as a tincture and as dried leaves, flowers, or roots, mullein can be used as an inhalant or taken as a tea.

Caution: Do not take mullein if you are nursing or if you have a history of cancer. Consult your doctor first; the tannin in mullein may be carcinogenic. Do not ingest the seeds; they are toxic.

GOLDENSEAL
(Hydrastis canadensis)

This thoroughly American herb, also known as orange root and ground raspberry, was discovered and widely used by early Native Americans, especially the Cherokee, as a general tonic and to dry up nasal and chest congestion. Its popularity then spread like wildfire among American settlers and immigrants, and it became the most frequently used herb in patent medicines. So frequently was it used and so highly was it prized, that by the turn of the twentieth century, it had been harvested nearly to extinction.

Today it remains a protected and expensive herb, but also a highly effective one. Its Greek name *hydrastis* means "to act on water" and refers to the root's superb ability—via its main chemical ingredient, the alkaloid hydrastine—to dry up the secretions of overactive mucous membranes in the chest, nose, throat, and sinuses. Goldenseal has proven anti-inflammatory and antibacterial properties. It also appears to act as a broad-spectrum antibiotic and is somewhat stimulating to the immune system. Thus it is often prescribed for throat, ear, gum, and sinus infections.

The dried root is available in herb, capsule, and tincture forms.

Caution: Do not use goldenseal without consulting a physician if you have heart disease, diabetes, glaucoma, high blood pressure, or if you have had a stroke.

FEVER, CHILLS, AND BODY ACHES

Fever, chills, and the body aches that accompany them respond best to herbs such as boneset, elder, and yarrow, among others, called diaphoretics. These are warming herbs that induce perspiration, stimulate blood circulation, and help break fevers. Most of these herbs also have some anti-inflammatory and analgesic properties that can help soothe and reduce the swelling of inflamed mucous membranes and relieve general aches and pains.

BONESET
(Eupatorium perfoliatum)

Boneset, also called sweat plant, feverwort, and Indian sage, was first used by Native Americans to treat colds, fevers, and body aches. News of boneset's healing properties soon spread among early American settlers, and by the 1800s boneset was the most popular of the patent folk medicines for all fever-producing illnesses and for aches and pains. Its common name has nothing to do with setting bones, but rather with its effectiveness in treating breakbone fever (also called dengue or blackwater fever), an acute viral infection carried by mosquitoes and characterized by high fever and severe joint pain.

Today, herbalists still consider boneset one of the best fever breakers as well as an effective analgesic for all types of muscle and joint pain—especially those of the flu, arthritis, and rheumatism.

Available as dried herb (leaves and flowers) and as a tincture, boneset is prescribed for short-term treatment of fever, colds, flu, coughs, and upper respiratory congestion. Boneset has a very bitter taste that you can mask with the addition of lemon and honey.

Caution: Only use the dried herb. Fresh boneset contains a toxic chemical called tremerol that can cause vomiting, rapid breathing, and at high doses, possibly coma and death. Do not take boneset for more than two weeks. If you have a history of alcoholism or liver problems, consult your herbalist before taking boneset; it is toxic to the liver.

ELDER
(Sambucus nigra)

Also called sambucus, sweet elder, and elderberry (elderberry wine is an old and famous folk drink), the small elder tree has a long history in treating infections with fever, at least as far back as the early Greeks who named it sambuca for an ancient stringed instrument called the sackbut. (The branches of the tree were used to make whistles and flutes.) In later centuries the elder was both feared and revered. Some cultures believed the tree harbored ghosts and symbolized death and suffering; two old Christian myths promulgated the belief that the elder was both the tree from which Judas hung himself and the tree used to make Christ's cross. Other cultures venerated the elder, planting it near their homes because of its mythical protective powers. Even today in some European countries, people are known to nod their heads in respect when passing an elder tree.

Those who revered the plant had good reason to do so. All parts of the elder—flower, barks, leaves, and roots—have medicinal properties. Besides being a confirmed diaphoretic and thus extremely effective in treating fever, elder is also rich in vitamins A, B, and C and is an excellent source of the plant pigment anthocyanin that has immune-stimulating properties. Current studies also seem to suggest that elder has antiviral and antibacterial properties, making it an excellent cold and flu fighter.

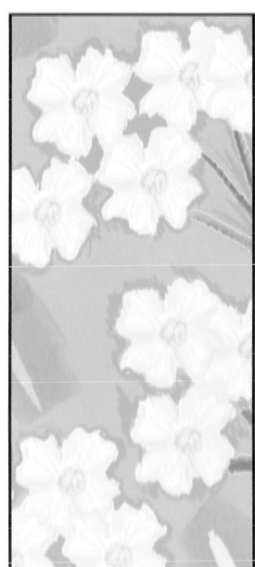

M i g h t y   H e r b a l

COLD AND FLU TEA

Steep 1 teaspoon each of peppermint, yarrow, and thyme in a generous cup of hot water. Drink three to four cups a day to help relieve the fever, aches, congestion, and inflammation related to colds and flus.

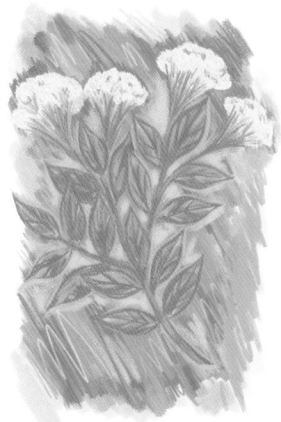

ELDER
(Sambucus nigra)

Taken internally for fevers, colds, and flus, elder is readily available as a tea (alone or with peppermint and yarrow) and in capsule, tincture, and dried herb forms. Follow your practitioner's or the manufacturer's directions.

YARROW
(Achillea millefolium)

As noted in Chapter 1, yarrow is an excellent wound healer, pain reliever, and anti-inflammatory; but it is also a proven diaphoretic that is most effective in treating colds and flus with fever. The leaves, stems, and flower tops contain salicylic acid—the same ingredient found in aspirin—that accounts for much of yarrow's fever-reducing and pain-relieving actions. The herb is also mildly sedating.

Yarrow is commercially available as a prepared tea and as dried herb. Like its cousin boneset, yarrow is quite bitter in taste. Adding honey and lemon to your tea can mask this taste.

Caution: If you are allergic to ragweed, you may be allergic to yarrow. Do not take yarrow with aspirin or with other herbs containing salicylic acid, such as white willow. Do not give yarrow to children.

SORE THROAT AND HEADACHE

The sore throat and aching head so characteristic of colds and the flu are due largely to inflammation of the mucous membranes in the throat and nose and to congestion in the nose and sinuses. Herbs that are anti-inflammatory, emollient, and astringent will reduce inflammation, soothe infected membranes, and help dry up congestion. When fever is present and infection is suspected, diaphoretic and antibacterial herbs are called for. Besides the herbs covered under "Fever, Chills, and Body Aches," the following are two of the best herbs for treating the sore throat and headache of colds and flu.

MYRRH
(Commiphora molmol)

Myrrh, an oil found in the bark of certain shrubs, has been esteemed for centuries as an exotic perfume and incense and is often mentioned in the Bible and ancient Greek and Arabic writings. The myrrh tree grows wild in Arabia, and its name derives from mur, the old Hebrew and Arabic word for bitter, from which the name "Mary" and all its many variations also come.

The gum resin made from myrrh oil has been equally prized for its potent healing effects. Myrrh has astringent, diaphoretic, and antiseptic properties, making it an excellent treatment for sore throats and aching heads where congestion is also present. Myrrh also reduces fevers and helps fight infections, primarily because of its antiseptic properties. However, recent research suggests that myrrh also stimulates the production of infection-fighting white blood cells and thus may be a natural antibiotic as well.

Herbalists prescribe myrrh for throat infections, sinusitis, chest congestion, asthma, coughs, and colds. For sore throats, myrrh is most often prescribed as a gargle. It is available in capsule, tincture, and powdered herb forms and may also be found in toothpastes and mouthwashes.

Caution: Use myrrh only on a short-term basis and do not exceed your practitioner's recommended doses. An overdose may cause a violent laxative action, vomiting, kidney problems, or accelerated heartbeat. Do not use if you suspect you are pregnant or are trying to conceive; myrrh is believed to have a stimulating effect on the uterus.

SLIPPERY ELM
(Ulmus fulva)

The FDA calls slippery elm a good demulcent (emollient) or soothing agent, and herbalists traditionally prescribe it both for sore throats and for upset stomachs. Slippery elm's active healing ingredient—3-methyl-galactose—is found in the smooth, slippery white inner bark, whose mucilaginous cells expand into a spongy mass when mixed with water.

Also known as red elm, slippery elm is additionally prescribed for coughs and congestion. It is available in capsule, tea, and powdered herb form.

ITCHY AND IRRITATED EYES

Red, itchy, running, sore, and irritated eyes are one of the hallmark symptoms of hay fever and very often accompany colds, flu, and sinus infections as well. There are many fine over-the-counter eye washes and drops that temporarily soothe itchy, irritated eyes, but none is as effective and broad-based a healer as eyebright.

EYEBRIGHT
(Euphrasia officinalis)

Eyebright is an outstanding example of why the medieval medical belief in the "Doctrine of Signatures" remained so popular for so long (but was ultimately proven wrong). The mainstay of that belief was the notion that how a plant looked was a clue to its medicinal use. Thus a plant with kidney-shaped leaves was believed to be good for kidney ailments.

Regretfully—and sometimes disastrously—that notion wasn't always true. But

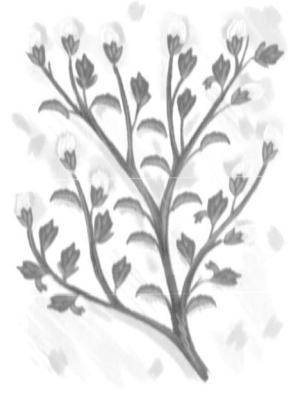

EYEBRIGHT
(Euphrasia officinalis)

The Eyes Have It . . .

Itchy, irritated eyes are not only hallmarks of colds and allergies, they are also painful reminders that we spend too much time indoors, in artificial air and light, doing repetitive tasks which tax our vision. When we do get outdoors, polluted air, damaging ultraviolet light, and waves of noxious carbon monoxide put a mighty strain on delicate eye tissue. We rarely think about nourishing our eyes the way we nourish our bodies, but we should: We need them for a lifetime. To nourish your eyes, make sure you get plenty of VITAMIN C-rich foods every day (oranges, grapefruits, strawberries, and broccoli, for example). Vitamin C helps restore the collagen (fluid) balance in eye tissue and lowers inner-eye pressure. Eat fresh HUCKLEBERRIES or BLUEBERRIES daily (in season) or drink a daily cup of huckleberry tea. This herb also helps maintain collagen balance, prevents the breakdown of vitamin C, improves poor night vision, and relieves eye strain. Also be sure to regularly eat foods or take supplements which contain VITAMIN B$_1$ (thiamin) and the minerals CHROMIUM and ZINC. Deficiencies of all three nutrients are associated with glaucoma and other chronic eye problems.

when it comes to eyebright, the appearance of the herb is very much related to its healing properties. The red spots on the white or purple flowers of this wild-growing plant seem to resemble bloodshot eyes. And since the Middle Ages, herbalists have in fact successfully prescribed eyebright—an anti-inflammatory, mild astringent, and infection fighter—for eyes that are itchy, red, and runny from hay fever, other allergies, colds, or conjunctivitis. Available in dried herb, capsule, and tincture form, eyebright is mostly prescribed as a lotion for the eyes. However, many herbalists believe that drinking eyebright as a tea can improve poor eyesight. It is also prescribed for internal use to treat nasal congestion, coughs, sinusitis, and allergies.

UPSET STOMACH, NAUSEA, AND VOMITING

All of Chapter 5 ("Calming an Upset Stomach") is devoted to herbs that treat various ailments of the stomach. But for the upset stomach, nausea, and vomiting that may accompany colds and almost always attend the flu, here are two common herbs that are uncommonly helpful in settling the stomach.

CINNAMON BARK
(*Cinnamomum verum; C. zeylanicum*)

Western cinnamon bark is prescribed for a variety of ailments, but most notably for stomach disorders, diarrhea (for which it is often taken in warm milk), and abdominal discomfort. It can also stimulate a poor appetite. Chinese cinnamon or cassia bark (*C. cassia*), a much stronger version of Western cinnamon and a potent stimulant, is native to China and Burma. Besides being prescribed for nausea and vomiting, Chinese cinnamon, which is increasingly popular in the West, may also be prescribed for impotence and delayed menstruation.

Cinnamon bark is available as fresh or dried, powdered herb, in commercially prepared teas (alone or in combination with other herbs), and in pill and tincture forms. Follow your practitioner's or the manufacturer's directions.

Caution: Large doses of cinnamon can cause changes in breathing, dilation of blood vessels, and convulsions. Do not use cinnamon when there is fever, inflammation, or bleeding.

MARSHMALLOW
(Althaea officinalis)

For most of us at the turn of the twenty-first century, the thought of marshmallows brings back memories of warm campfire nights and the gooey, white confections we toasted on the ends of sticks and branches. But for centuries people in Europe and the Middle East ate wild-growing marshmallows when their crops failed.

Also known as sweet weed and Althea (from the Greek altho, meaning "to heal"), marshmallow is still recognized as a wilderness forage food, but herbalists prize it more for its many therapeutic benefits. Because of its high mucilage content, marshmallow tea is very soothing to inflamed mucous membranes of the stomach and intestine and is often prescribed for gastritis, colitis, constipation, and peptic ulcers.

Marshmallow is available as bulk dried herb and in capsule, tincture, and teas. Unlike most other herbal teas, marshmallow tea is considered more potent when cold. After making a tea, refrigerate it until completely cool.

More
Helpful Advice
VIRUSES AND BACTERIA AND POLLEN . . . OH MY!

Your grandmother probably said it first, and it's still true today: An ounce of prevention is far better than spending a week in bed with the flu, refereeing a houseful of preschoolers with colds, or heralding the first Spring weekend with a big, red nose. Developing a strong immune system is your absolute best defense against viral, bacterial, and allergen invasions. Immune-boosting herbs such as echinacea, goldenseal, and garlic will not only prevent many infections and allergy attacks, they'll also shorten the duration of the ones that sneak by you. You also need to get plenty of vitamins C, A, and B-complex, together with the minerals zinc and copper. These are the super supplements that work hand-in-hand with a healthy diet to help the body ward off attacks. Drink lots of water, get plenty of rest, and—as selfish as it sounds—avoid infected or allergy-triggering people, places, and things.

Maintaining
Healthy Skin

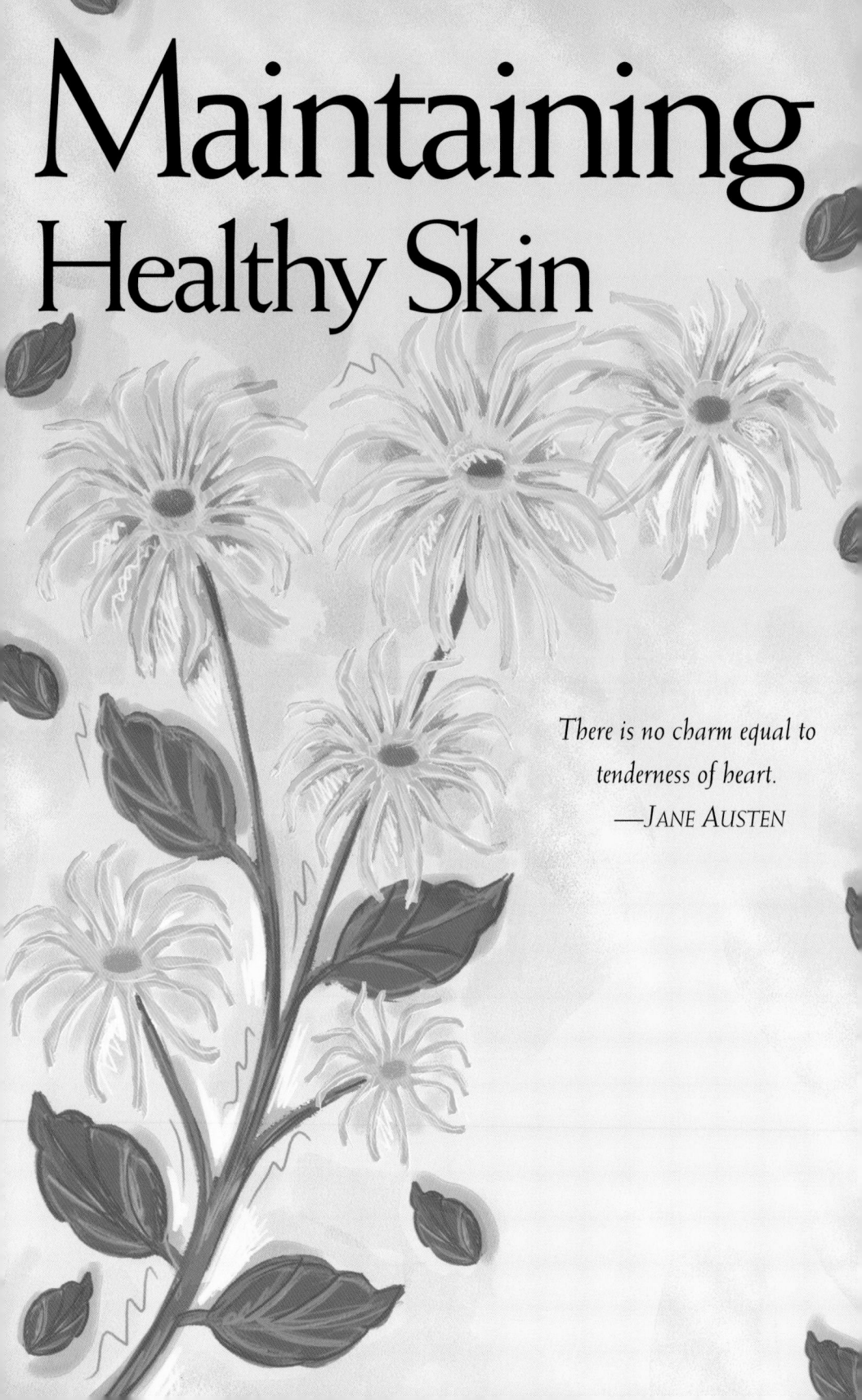

There is no charm equal to
tenderness of heart.
—JANE AUSTEN

MORE THAN SKIN DEEP

Skin, the largest organ of our body, is also the most vulnerable to attack from just about every offending corner. Sun, wind, cold, heat, water, fire, illness, allergens, viruses, bacteria, insects, food, pollutants, cosmetics, and time all conspire to damage, weaken, or infect the skin.

Not surprisingly, treating skin ailments was among the first uses humankind found for medicinal plants. In fact, so many plant herbs are useful in treating the skin that it is difficult to highlight just a few of the best herbs for treatment—as we do here.

For one thing, there is much overlap among the therapeutic properties of these herbs. Many herbs that are effective in treating eczema (or dermatitis), for example, which is essentially an allergy-based ailment, are also good for treating psoriasis, which is an autoimmune disease. Wherever an herb may be helpful for more than one condition, we point this out, regardless of the category in which the herb is listed. So it is useful in this chapter especially to read through all the herb entries.

The other problem with identifying specific herbs for the skin is the fact that skin ailments are unique to an individual's biochemical makeup and are notoriously hard to treat. What works for one acne sufferer may not work for another. Trying different herbs to see what works best for your special case is often the rule, not the exception.

Self-treating skin problems, therefore, is an area where working with a qualified herbal practitioner will be most beneficial, especially if you are new to herbs. The practitioner will likely treat any skin ailment in two distinct ways. First, an attempt will be made to identify the underlying internal cause of the ailment and treat it internally with the most appropriate multitherapeutic herb. Second, herbs that provide quick and soothing symptomatic relief will also be prescribed, often as topical applications, but also internally as teas and decoctions.

Let's look first at the herbs commonly used to treat underlying conditions or illnesses associated with skin problems. Then we'll move on to specific herbs for specific ailments.

HERBAL TONICS FOR THE SKIN

Many herbalists believe that most skin ailments have their origins in systemic weaknesses, toxicity, and illnesses of the body's blood, circulatory and digestive systems, and organs such as the kidneys and liver, both of which are responsible for cleaning the blood and eliminating toxins from the body. Herbs that are "alterative" are frequently prescribed when underlying weakness or toxicity is suspected. Alterative herbs enrich, detoxify, and normalize the blood, repair infected or weak tissues, and strengthen and support organs and organ function.

Because of their role in detoxifying and eliminating waste products, the liver and kidneys are often the primary targets of alterative herbs. Echinacea is an excellent example of an alterative herb that targets the liver. When the kidneys are the suspected culprits in a skin condition, alteratives with diuretic properties, such as dandelion, may be prescribed. When infection—viral or bacterial—may also be a contributing factor, herbs that are antibiotic, antibacterial, or immune stimulating may be added to the mix. Echinacea and astragalus are examples of such herbs.

(We will look again at these herbs in more depth in Chapter 7, "Strengthening Your Immune System.")

Here are four of the best alterative herbs for treating some of the underlying causes of skin ailments.

ANGELICA SINENSIS/ DONG QUAI
(Angelica sinensis)

Also known as Chinese angelica root and *tang gui*, angelica—long a staple among Chinese herbalists—is increasingly used in the West. While Asian and some Western herbalists prescribe angelica primarily for gynecological complaints (see Chapter 6), it is a renowned general tonic that balances (tonifies) the entire body. Saponin, one of its primary ingredients, is believed responsible for this balancing effect. Angelica detoxifies the blood, promotes optimal organ function (especially reproductive and digestive organs), supports a strong circulatory system, and stimulates energy and healing. It also has sedating, pain-relieving, and laxative properties.

It has traditionally been taken internally for poor blood circulation, possible anemia, abscesses, boils, and sores. It may also be useful in the treatment of acne, eczema, and psoriasis.

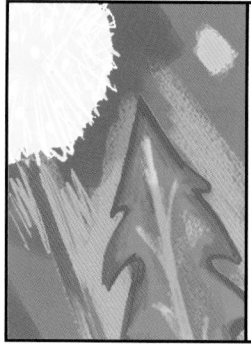

F a s t   R e l i e f   f o r

INSECT BITES

Squeeze some sap from a dandelion stem and rub directly on the bite for a soothing and healing effect. Nettle lotion or ointment (see Chapter 2, p. 21) also relieves the swelling and pain of insect bites.

The medicinal root is available in bulk dried herb, capsules, tincture, and tonic forms at health food stores and Asian markets and pharmacies. You should avoid the dried herb if it is dry or has a greenish-brown cross-section.

Caution: Angelica sinensis is a uterine stimulant and a laxative. Do not take it if you suspect you are pregnant, or if you are trying to conceive. Do not take it if you have diarrhea or bloating. Consult a practitioner instead.

ASTRAGALUS/MILK-VETCH ROOT
(Astragalus membranaceus)

The perennial plant astragalus, or milk vetch root, has a long history of use among Asian herbalists, who know it as *huang qi* (or *ch'i*), and it is increasingly used by Western herbalists as well. The polysaccharides in astragalus are believed partly responsible for the herb's superb immune-stimulating properties, which are the subject of considerable AIDS and cancer research. (We also discuss astragalus's antiviral and antitumor properties in Chapters 2 and 7.)

Like angelica sinensis, astragalus generally strengthens the body, nourishes the blood, promotes tissue repair, stimulates the metabolism, and increases energy. Recent research also has shown that astragalus fights bacteria and detoxifies the gastrointestinal system.

It is traditionally prescribed for chronic weakness and fatigue, diarrhea, blood abnormalities, and acute skin conditions where there is swelling, pus formation, and/or chronic ulceration. It may therefore be useful in the treatment of acne, boils, eczema, hives, and psoriasis.

Astragalus is available as a prepared tea and in tincture, capsule, and dried herb form.

DANDELION
(Taraxacum officinale)

Dandelion's long history of medicinal use includes its therapeutic role as a tonifying diuretic that adds the essential mineral potassium to the body (rather than removing it as most diuretics do). Dandelion is an especially effective tonic for cleansing the blood, liver, and kidneys and has been prescribed for internal use in treating skin rashes, acne, boils, eczema, and poison ivy and oak. (Externally, its sap is rubbed on insect bites and warts.) It also has cardiotonic properties that we discuss more in the next chapter.

Dandelion is available in tinctures, prepared teas, capsules, and dried or fresh leaves or roots. The fresh leaves, rich in vitamins A and C, iron, and minerals, may also be added to salads.

ECHINACEA
(Echinacea purpurea, E. pallida, E. angustifolia)

Perhaps the most talked about and researched herb today, echinacea is a superb alterative and immune stimulant with both antiviral and antibacterial actions. This makes it an excellent and broad-based internal and external herbal treatment for a variety of skin ailments. (We discuss echinacea's other immune-stimulating and antiviral properties in greater detail in Chapters 2 and 7.)

Internally, echinacea is prescribed most frequently to cleanse and tonify the blood, strengthen and detoxify the kidneys and liver, and stimulate the immune system to fight underlying viral and bacterial infections. Externally, it has been prescribed (in tinctures and ointments) for boils, abscesses, insect bites and stings, hives, eczema, and cold sores (herpes simplex).

Echinacea is available in tea, capsule, tincture, ointment, and dried bulk form. Follow your practitioner's or the manufacturer's directions.

Caution: You should not take echinacea continuously for more than a few weeks. Consult a qualified practitioner if you feel you need to continue treatment beyond that. Do not take echinacea if you have an autoimmue disorder.

HERBAL REMEDIES FOR SKIN AILMENTS

ACNE

The bane of adolescents and many adults, too, acne is an all too common inflammatory skin condition characterized by blackheads, whiteheads, pimples, inflamed and pus-filled nodules and cysts, and sometimes deep, infected, craterlike lesions in the skin. Acne may appear on the face, neck, shoulders, chest, and back and if not treated adequately, it can result in scarring and disfigurement—although thankfully this is the exception, not the rule.

Acne occurs most frequently with hormonal changes, but may also be tied to genetic predisposition, nutrition, stress, and environmental pollutants. Alterative herbs that detoxify the blood and nourish and support the liver have been used with great success for treating acne internally and externally. Two of these are cleavers and yellow dock.

Nothing worth doing is completed in our lifetime; therefore, we must be saved by hope. Nothing true or beautiful or good makes complete sense in any immediate context of history; therefore, we must be saved by faith. Nothing we do, however virtuous, can be accomplished alone; therefore, we are saved by love.

—REINHOLD NIEBUHR

CLEAVERS
(Galium aparine)

Commonly known as clivers (because the stems cling or "cleave" to clothes and other surfaces) and goosegrass (because geese are fond of grazing on it), cleavers has been used medicinally at least since the ancient Greeks who called it *philanthropon* ("love-man") because of the plant's clinging tendency.

Among folk herbalists, cleavers was used to treat wounds, urinary infections, and chronic "dry" skin conditions such as psoriasis. Today the herb is prescribed internally for a range of infections that involve the lymphatic system (tonsillitis, for example); for urinary infections; and for acne, eczema, and psoriasis. Cleavers is a powerful alterative and lymphatic tonic. As an alterative, it cleanses the blood and aids in the elimination of toxins from the body; it particularly supports the kidneys. As a lymphatic tonic, it targets swollen and infected glands and promotes drainage.

Available in dried herb, capsule, tincture, and ointment forms, cleavers is prescribed for internal use mostly as a tea or tincture. Externally, an ointment made with cleavers may be applied directly to dry, scaling, and irritated skin. Follow your practitioner's or the manufacturer's directions.

YELLOW DOCK
(*Rumex crispus*)

Also known as curly or curled dock and rumex, yellow dock has a long history of use by European and American herbalists who most frequently prescribed the medicinal root for what they called "obstinate" skin ailments—eczema, ringworm, and scabies among others. (One of yellow dock's primary ingredients, rumicin, is believed to destroy parasites.) Yellow dock is an alterative that nourishes and supports the liver, gall bladder, and colon (it is also prescribed for constipation), and is a fine astringent and blood tonic that "cools" and detoxifies blood.

Available in dried herb, capsule, and tincture forms, yellow dock is frequently prescribed for internal use to treat acne, psoriasis, eczema, and other skin ailments

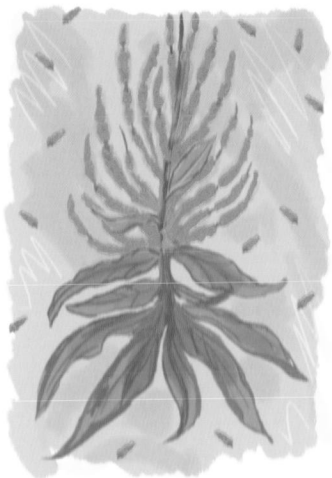

Y E L L O W   D O C K
(*Rumex crispus*)

with chronic irritation. Externally, it can be applied in poultices and ointments directly to inflamed and infected swellings and sores. Follow your practitioner's or the manufacturer's directions.

Caution: Excessive use of yellow dock can cause nausea.

ATHLETE'S FOOT AND OTHER FUNGAL INFECTIONS

Athlete's foot and other fungal infections, such as ringworm and the infamous "jock" itch, are caused by microscopic organisms that usually live happily on the surface of the skin and cause no problems. Under certain conditions, however, these organisms may start to grow into pesky, painful, red, and infectious lesions and blisters. Hot, moist weather combined with skin that rarely gets a chance to "breathe" (go without shoes or sneakers), existing skin irritations or cuts, and some underlying illnesses may all conspire to create fungal infections.

Effective herbal treatments for fungal infections include the topical use of essential oils from herbs that are antimicrobials and have antibacterial, infection-fighting properties. Two of these are myrrh and tea (ti) tree. Internal treatments include herbs with proven antifungal action, pau d'arco.

MYRRH
(Commiphora molmol)

In Chapter 2, we discuss in great detail the internal use of myrrh for treating some of the symptoms of colds and flu. Myrrh's antibacterial and infection-fighting properties are found in the essential oil of the tree's bark. This oil, which is made into a tincture, is a very strong astringent, and for topical application it is often combined with other herbs such as calendula and witch hazel, which are milder astringents and have cooling, soothing properties. Myrrh may also be combined with almond oil.

Myrrh mixtures are applied topically to the irritated skin, lesions, and blisters of athlete's foot and other fungal infections. Myrrh oil is also prescribed as a topical application for insect bites, cold sores, and psoriasis. Research indicates that the herb fights infection by stimulating the production of white blood cells. It is readily available as powdered herb and as a tincture.

Caution: Use only small amounts of any essential oil. Large amounts of myrrh may cause a violent laxative action, profuse sweating, vomiting, kidney problems, or accelerated heartbeat. This normally applies only to the internal use of myrrh, but if any of these symptoms do occur with topical application, call your doctor immediately. Also consult your physician or herbalist before starting use if you have kidney disease.

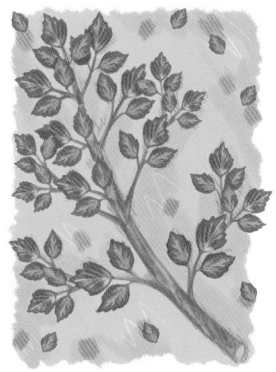

M Y R R H
(Commiphora molmol)

PAU D'ARCO
(Tabebuia impetiginosa)

Pau d'arco is the name of both the tree and the medicinal extract taken from the tree's bark. Long before modern science isolated some 20 of its chemical ingredients, pau d'arco was effectively used for hundreds of years by folk herbalists to treat bacterial, fungal, viral, and parasitic infections. Research indicates that pau d'arco appears to destroy infectious micro-organisms by increasing the supply of oxygen to cells.

Pau d'arco is applied externally for athlete's foot and yeast infections and taken as a tea or tincture for bacterial, fungal, viral, and parasitic infections. It is available in capsule, tincture, and dried bark form. To make a decoction at home, boil 1 tablespoon of dried bark in 2 to 3 cups of water for 10 to 15 minutes and strain. Drink 2 to 8 cups a day.

TEA (TI) TREE OIL
(Melaleuca alternifolia)

Ten years ago, tea tree oil, from a native tree of the Australian bottle brush species, was rarely seen in this country, although it was used in Europe in the early 1700s both internally (for tuberculosis and bronchitis) and externally (for rheumatism and tooth pain).

Now tea tree oil is widely available in a variety of forms and is sometimes endowed (incorrectly) with panacea-like properties for a wide range of ailments from colds and sinusitis, coughs and congestion, to sunburn and malaria, head lice and insect bites. In fact, tea tree oil—its most available form—is an excellent topical treatment for fungal infections, including athlete's foot, ring-worm, and thrush.

Research has shown that tea tree's antibiotic action is due primarily to a single ingredient, terpineol. The oil, which smells like nutmeg, is extracted from the leaves by steam distillation.

Tea tree is readily available as an oil and can be found with other ingredients in a variety of health and beauty products. (It is also used in flea shampoos.) Follow your practitioner's or the manufacturer's directions.

Caution: Use only small amounts of any essential oil. People with sensitive skin should dilute tea tree with a bland oil, such as vegetable or almond oil.

BOILS

Boils (also called carbuncles) are inflamed and pus-infected nodules caused by the staphylococcus bacteria. They appear as red, raised bumps that are tender and painful to the touch. Many herbalists believe these types of skin eruptions are related to poor liver functioning and underlying infection. Any of the general alteratives discussed earlier would make a fine, broad-based treatment if systemic weaknesses and infection are suspected. Echinacea is a good choice because

And God smiled again, And the rainbow appeared, And curled itself around his shoulder.
—JAMES WELDON JOHNSON,
GOD'S TROMBONES

of its special affinity for the liver. Two other alterative herbs have traditionally been used specifically to treat boils—blue flag and fenugreek.

BLUE FLAG
(Iris versicolor)

Also known as flag lily and liver lily, blue flag, a member of the iris family, is a powerful, infection-fighting alterative that appears to target the liver directly, helping to stimulate sluggish liver function and increase the elimination of toxic substances, especially where infection is present. The dried root and leaves were used extensively by Native Americans for gastrointestinal problems and as a diuretic, and the popularity of the plant spread among early American settlers, who used the herb for skin diseases, blood problems, rheumatism, and syphilis.

Today blue flag is mainly prescribed for "eruptive" skin conditions, such as boils and acne, and is usually taken internally as a tea. Blue flag is available as dried herb.

Caution: Use dried root only; the fresh root may be toxic. Blue flag is a powerful alterative and should be taken for only a short period of time. We recommend that you work with a qualified practitioner if you use this herb. Do not harvest blue flag yourself. It is very similar in appearance to sweet flag or calamus (*Acorus calamus*), which has vastly different therapeutic properties. (It is used primarily to treat flatulence.) Questions also have been raised about sweet flag's possible carcinogenicity.

FENUGREEK
(Trigonella foenum-graecum)

Often thought of only as a culinary herb or fodder for cattle, fenugreek—also known as

Greek hay—has a long history of medicinal use among Asian and Western herbalists and can be traced back to Ancient Egypt and Greece.

It has been prescribed internally to treat general weakness and debilitation, poor appetite, constipation, and abdominal pain and discomfort. In Chinese herbal medicine, it is considered one of the finest yang tonics; that is, one of the warming tonics that detoxify and nourish the blood and have a special affinity for the kidneys. Externally, fenugreek is frequently used in compresses and poultices to treat boils, hives, and similar skin eruptions.

The dried ripe seeds of the plant contain most of its medicinal properties and may be made into a tea for internal use or applied topically in a compress or poultice.

Caution: Fenugreek is a uterine stimulant. Do not take it if you suspect you are pregnant or if you are trying to conceive.

Even in America, the Indian summer of life should be a little sunny and a little sad, like the season, and infinite in wealth and depth of tone—but never hustled.
—HENRY BROOKS ADAMS

COLD SORES (HERPES SIMPLEX)

Cold sores are small, fluid-filled blisters that appear around the mouth and are caused by the herpes simplex virus. Most people are first infected with herpes simplex when they are quite young, and after that first infection the virus usually remains dormant. Cold sores may be triggered later in life, however, by illness, stress, immune deficiency, menstruation, or pregnancy. Additionally, some people seem prone to chronic outbreaks.

Any of the general alteratives described earlier may be used as supportive therapy for a cold sore outbreak. Myrrh oil may be applied topically to relieve pain and enhance healing. Two other tonic herbs have been used specifically for the herpes simplex virus. For genital herpes, consult a qualified medical practitioner.

GENTIAN/YELLOW GENTIAN
(Gentiana lutea)

This yellow-flowered perennial is probably named for Gentius, the Greek king of Illyria circa 180 B.C. who is supposed to have discovered it. Gentian has long been considered the most bitter of the "bitter" herbs. And bitter herbs "cool" inflammatory infections, stimulate the appetite, promote good digestion, and dry up moist and oozing skin ailments, such as cold sores. Gentian is also an alterative used to treat general debility and weakness (conditions that may precipitate an outbreak of cold sores) and to strengthen liver function (which is critical to clearing infectious toxins from the blood).

Taken internally, gentian is available as a tincture and as dried root.

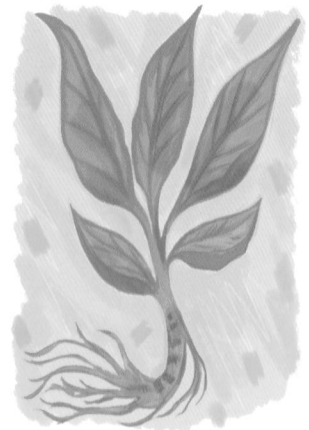

**GENTIAN/
YELLOW GENTIAN**
(Gentiana lutea)

Caution: Do not use if you suspect you are pregnant or are trying to conceive. Consult a practitioner before use if you have high blood pressure.

SARSAPARILLA
(Similax officinalis)

More popularly known as a soft drink flavoring, sarsaparilla has a long history in treating chronic, systemic skin problems such as herpes and psoriasis. In fact, sarsaparonin, a primary chemical ingredient of sarsaparilla, is used in tablets to treat psoriasis.

Popularly known by a variety of common names—wild sarsaparilla, wild spikenard, and American sarsaparilla—the medicinal root of sarsaparilla is a warming alterative and diuretic that detoxifies the blood, supports the lymphatic system, and aids the kidneys in removing toxic substances from the body.

Sarsaparilla is available as dried herb and tea. For cold sores and psoriasis, it may be taken internally as a tea or applied topically in a warm compress.

ECZEMA AND HIVES

Eczema—also called dermatitis—is a very itchy, red rash that can be accompanied by scaling, scabbing, crusting, peeling, and oozing. With scratching and other irritations, bleeding and infection may occur. Eczema is often an allergic reaction to something that has been touched; then it is called contact dermatitis. It may also be triggered by hay fever and other internal allergies, as well as by stress, certain food products, and heat.

Hives, also called urticaria, are almost always caused by allergic reactions—internal or external in origin—to a vast array of potential allergens. Hives appear, usually in clusters, as raised bumps or welts that are red, itchy, and hot. They may appear and disappear quite quickly, often in just a day, but often reoccur if triggered by the original allergen. Isolated outbreaks of hives are common for many people and can be self-treated. Some hive outbreaks, however, such as those triggered by an insect bite, can be life threatening and must be quickly treated by medical personnel.

Although the specific causes of eczema and hives are often hard to pinpoint, many herbs have been used both internally and topically to relieve these skin conditions, support the

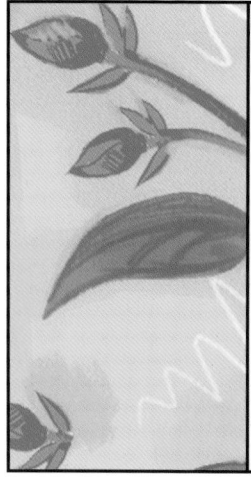

body during outbreaks, prevent secondary infection, and provide symptomatic relief. Here are a few of the best.

FIGWORT
(*Scrophularia nodosa*)

Figwort—also known as throatwort, carpenter's square, and scrofula plant—is another of the warming, blood-purifying, and diuretic alteratives that have a long and successful track record in treating skin diseases caused by underlying infection or weakness. Again, this herb specifically targets the kidneys and liver, together with the lymphatic (glandular) system. In fact, scrofula is a medical term for swollen glands, and the plant gets its botanical name from the fact that knobby protrusions on the root look like enlarged and infected glands.

Here is an herb that has been prescribed almost exclusively for skin diseases. In the Middle Ages it was used for treating wounds, gangrene, abscesses, swellings, and burns. More recently it has been increasingly prescribed for eczema and psoriasis, and for acute skin conditions with itching and irritation, such as hives.

Available as a tincture and in dried herb form, figwort is most often taken internally as a tea.

Caution: Figwort is also a cardiotonic and heart stimulant, although not at all toxic as are some cardiotonics, such as foxglove, which is the source for digitalis. We strongly recommend, however, that you take figwort under the care of a qualified practitioner, particularly if you have tachycardia (an overly rapid heartbeat) or any other heart condition.

FUMITORY
(*Fumaria officinalis*)

Fumitory's poetic common name—earth smoke—has been variously explained as a reference to the hazy, gray-blue appearance of the leaves that look like smoke when viewed from a distance and by the ancient belief that the plant was mysteriously born from the steamy, smoky vapors of the earth, rather than from seed, and could ward off evil spirits.

Since the days of ancient Rome, fumitory has been prized as a blood-purifying alternative tonic with a special affinity for strengthening the liver. It also acts as a gentle diuretic and laxative and combines well with cleavers and figwort in teas. Fumitory fell out of favor as a medicinal herb for some time and was wrongly labeled as poisonous in some herbal manuals. Available as dried herb, tea, and tincture, fumitory is now being prescribed more frequently as an internal and external treatment for acne, eczema, and scaly skin conditions.

Caution: Fumitory has sedating and hypnotic properties when taken in large doses or over a long period of time. If you plan to take it for more than a week, work with a qualified herbal practitioner.

OREGON MOUNTAIN GRAPE
(*Mahonia aquifolium*)

Also known as mountain grape, this is a relatively new herb in the West, first introduced in Europe in the early 1800s as an ornamental shrub. The valuable medicinal properties of mountain grape's root and rhizome were soon discovered, however, and the herb is now prized as a potent tonic alterative with laxative effects that is equally prescribed for digestive problems and for hard-to-treat chronic and scaly skin conditions such as eczema and psoriasis. It has also been successfully used to treat acne and herpes simplex.

Herbalists often combine mountain grape with cleavers and yellow dock for a potent healing tea for the skin. The herb is available as dried root and as a tincture.

DRY OR SUNBURNED SKIN

Dry or sunburned skin is damaged skin that begs for moisture, soothing emollients, and relief from pain and itching. Aloe and calendula are two of the best herbal skin soothers.

ALOE
(*Aloe barbadensis*)

The translucent gel obtained from the inner leaves of the aloe plant is used externally to relieve minor burns, skin irritations, and infections. (Taken internally, aloe relieves stomach upsets.) Rich with polysaccharides that act as soothing emollients on damaged skin, aloe also reduces inflammation and redness.

Apply externally for minor burns, wounds, insect bites, rashes, sunburn, poison ivy, and acne. Aloe is available as a powder, fluid extract, bottled gel, or capsules. Follow your practitioner's or the manufacturer's directions.

For a soothing, healing herbal bath, add 1 to 2 cups of aloe gel to a warm bath to relieve sunburn, dry and itchy skin, eczema, or psoriasis.

Caution: If you have a gastrointestinal illness, consult an herbalist or your practitioner before taking aloe internally.

MARIGOLD/CALENDULA
(*Calendula officinalis*)

The common marigold is the most famous flower of the calendula family, whose uses as a medicine can be traced back to ancient Egypt and Greece, where it was used for medicinal, culinary, and cosmetic purposes. During the Middle Ages, calendula was a traditional treatment for smallpox, measles, and insect bites.

A natural antiseptic and anti-inflammatory agent—and an alterative herb that promotes the secretion of bile—calendula also has soothing properties that, together with its anti-inflammatory and antiseptic actions, make it one of the best herbs for treating burns, wounds, skin abrasions, eruptions, and infections. Calendula has also been used successfully to treat eczema and acne. The herb's healing power appears to come

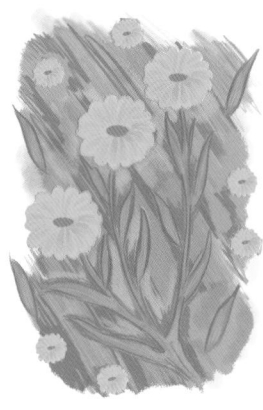

MARIGOLD/CALENDULA
(Calendula officinalis)

from components known as terpenes, which also have a sedating effect and may help in the management of accompanying pain.

Calendula is commercially available in lotions, ointments, creams, oils, tinctures, and as fresh or dried leaves and flowers. Follow your practitioner's or the manufacturer's advice.

PSORIASIS

This common skin disease is often classified as both hereditary and autoimmune in nature (a condition where an overactive immune system turns on itself). The rash, although not normally itchy, appears as red, painful-looking, raised lesions that develop silver-colored scales. The rash may be confined to a small area or it may cover large parts of the body. The condition itself is characterized by cycles of outbreak and remission that seem linked to stress, infection, and underlying systemic conditions, most particularly arthritis. For some individuals, the rash becomes disfiguring and disabling, causing emotional and physical problems. Psoriasis is notoriously unresponsive to medical interventions; there is no definitive treatment, although exposure to sunlight provides much relief for some sufferers.

Herbs may provide an avenue for both systemic treatment of underlying infection and weaknesses (any of the major alterative herbs discussed earlier would be useful) and symptomatic relief. Working with a qualified practitioner is a must. Two herbs that are frequently used for scaly skin conditions are Balm of Gilead and burdock.

BALM OF GILEAD
(Populus candicans)

This member of the poplar tree family, although not often listed in current herb books, has a history that stretches back to at least biblical times (it is referred to frequently in the Bible). Its flower buds—the medicinal part of the tree—were once reputed to have miraculous properties.

Also called poplar buds, the herb has antimicrobial (infection-fighting), wound-healing, and expectorant actions and is rich in natural pain relievers and soothing emollients that have a special affinity for the mucous membranes. Thus Balm of Gilead is frequently prescribed as an internal remedy for congestive coughs, sore throats, and laryngitis.

It is equally effective as an external treatment for rheumatic and arthritic pain and swelling, and for dry and scaly skin ailments, such as psoriasis.

Balm of Gilead is available as dried herb (the flower buds) and as a tincture. As a tincture it can be mixed with vegetable oil to make a topical application to spread on skin lesions. Because Balm of Gilead also is an astringent that can sometimes cause irritation, a soothing emollient herb such as calendula may be added to the mix.

BURDOCK/GREATER BURDOCK
(Arctium lappa)

Also known as beggar's buttons, lappa, and pig's rhubarb, burdock is famous for its tiny, hooked burrs that attach themselves to anything and everything—as anyone who has taken a walk through the woods with their dog can attest to.

Medicinally, burdock is just as famous and has long been prescribed for a wide range of illnesses. But it is especially valued as a treatment for stubborn, scaly skin ailments like psoriasis, especially when it is accompanied by arthritis or rheumatism. In fact, some herbal practitioners believe that long-term treatment with burdock tea taken internally may be the best and most effective, broad-based treatment for psoriasis. Burdock may also be applied topically to skin lesions for symptomatic relief.

Burdock is available as dried powder, slices of root, and tincture.

Caution: Burdock is a uterine stimulant. Do not use it if you suspect you are pregnant or if you are trying to conceive.

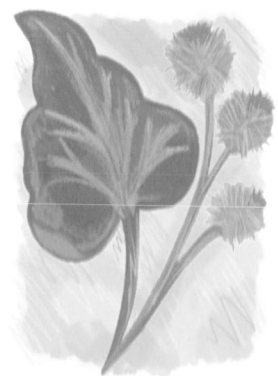

BURDOCK/GREATER
BURDOCK
(Arctium lappa)

POISON IVY AND POISON OAK

The red and itchy rash of poison ivy and poison oak is caused by a resin, urushiol, on the plants' leaves. Urushiol is a specific allergen, not a poison, which is why some people can roll in poison ivy and never get so much as a blotch, whereas other urushiol-sensitive people—who merely touch an animal or piece of clothing that's been in contact with the plants—develop a full-blown rash, complete with watery blisters and inflammation. Here are two great soothers of poison ivy and oak rashes. They are also good for sunburn, insect bites, and bee stings.

PLANTAIN HERB
(Plantago psyllium)

Psyllium—commonly known as plantain—is most famous for its seeds, which are rich in fiber, making it a safe, bulk-forming laxative. Thus the herb—whose other common names include pigweed, flea seed, and French psyllium—has long been used internally to treat constipation, diarrhea, hemorrhoids, and urinary problems. (See Chapter

6, "Calming an Upset Stomach," for a more detailed discussion of plantain.)

The leaves of the plantain have markedly different but just as valuable therapeutic properties. They promote cooling, astringent, and wound-healing action. Made into a tea or poultice, the crushed leaves have long been used to treat poison ivy and oak, bee stings, insect bites, wounds, warts, and most notably, hemorrhoids.

Fresh or dried, crushed plantain leaves may be made into a poultice and applied directly to the skin.

Caution: Plantain can cause allergic reactions in people who have allergies to dust or grasses. Call your doctor if you have an allergic reaction.

WITCH HAZEL
(Hamamelis virginiana)

This small tree, native to North America, owes its common name to an early association with witchcraft and to the fact that its forklike branches were used to search for water.

Native Americans first used the liquid extract from the bark of the tree as an eyewash,

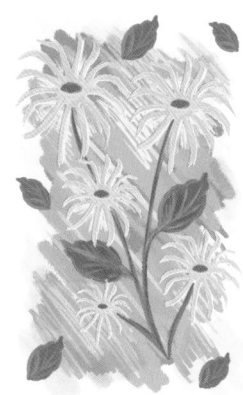

WITCH HAZEL
(Hamamelis virginiana)

pain reliever, and wound healer, all indications for which the herb is still used today.

Indeed, witch hazel is the most recognizable—and most commercially available—of the great herbs. It is a classic "cooling" herb with astringent and anti-inflammatory properties. The distilled witch hazel found in most homes is a perfect topical treatment for poison ivy and oak. (Undiluted, natural witch hazel extracts, however, are too astringent and can cause scarring.) Commercial witch hazel will help relieve itching and pain and reduce swelling and redness. It is also a soothing treatment for sunburn and insect bites.

Apply with cotton or on a cloth directly to affected skin.

WARTS

Warts are small, raised growths that look like tiny cauliflowers and appear most often on the hands and the soles of the feet, where they are called plantar warts. (Warts, which are contagious, are also common in the genital area, but these should be treated by a qualified medical practitioner.) Many warts go away without any treatment. Those that don't are infamous for being hard to get rid of. That's because a virus for which there is no effective cure causes warts. Topical applications—and some medical procedures, such as freezing—can temporarily remove warts, but they sometimes reappear. The oil or sap of some herbs may be helpful in removing common warts; the sap of the dandelion, discussed earlier, is a famous wart remover. Black walnut may be one of the few effective systemic remedies, and greater celandine is another famous topical application.

BLACK WALNUT
(Juglans nigra)

Black walnut's bark, leaves, fruit rind, and liquid extracts are prescribed by herbalists for fungal and parasitic infections, mouth sores, and warts. In fact, some research suggests that when taken internally and used over the long term, black walnut will help permanently eliminate warts. The herb is rich in tannins and iodine, which makes it an excellent antiseptic, and it is also believed to detoxify the blood.

Black walnut is available as tincture, extract, and dried herb (bark, leaves, and fruit rind). Follow your practitioner's advice for internal consumption of black walnut. For external use, rub the extract on the warts twice a day.

GREATER CELANDINE
(Chelidonium majus)

The Ancient Greek physician and botanist Dioscorides named the herb chelidonium after the Greek word *khelidon*, which means "swallow," supposedly because the plant blooms when the swallows return home.

Greater celandine's medicinal use can be traced back to Ancient Greece and Rome, where it was known as a hypnotic and purgative, but it was most widely used in the Middle Ages as a treatment for the plague and various blood ailments.

Available as fresh or dried herb for the treatment of intestinal problems, greater celandine can be poisonous when taken internally in too large a dose. Externally, however, greater celandine has enjoyed some success as a wart remover—the orange sap extracted from the leaves and stems has long been used as a topical application for warts. Check with a qualified practitioner for the correct way to use the herb.

Caution: Large doses of greater celandine taken internally are extremely toxic. Do not use internally.

More Helpful Advice
WATER, WATER, EVERYWHERE . . .

It's in our teeth, bones, blood, and cells; tissue, urine, fat, and perspiration; muscles, mucous, saliva, and skin. Water. On any given day, our body is filled to the brim with it—as much as 50 quarts of water, which we mostly take for granted. But if we lost even 8 or 9 quarts of it, we'd probably also lose our lives. That's how important water is to a well-functioning body. And with a loss of just 4 or 5 quarts, we're in danger: Our muscles begin to atrophy, our skin shrivels up, we become exhausted to the point of collapse, and our body's life-sustaining systems start to shut down. Water keeps our body cool; our skin supple; our blood, kidneys, liver, and intestines free of toxins and enriched with oxygen; our muscles strong; and our joints flexible. Do your body a favor and drink at least 8 glasses of water a day.

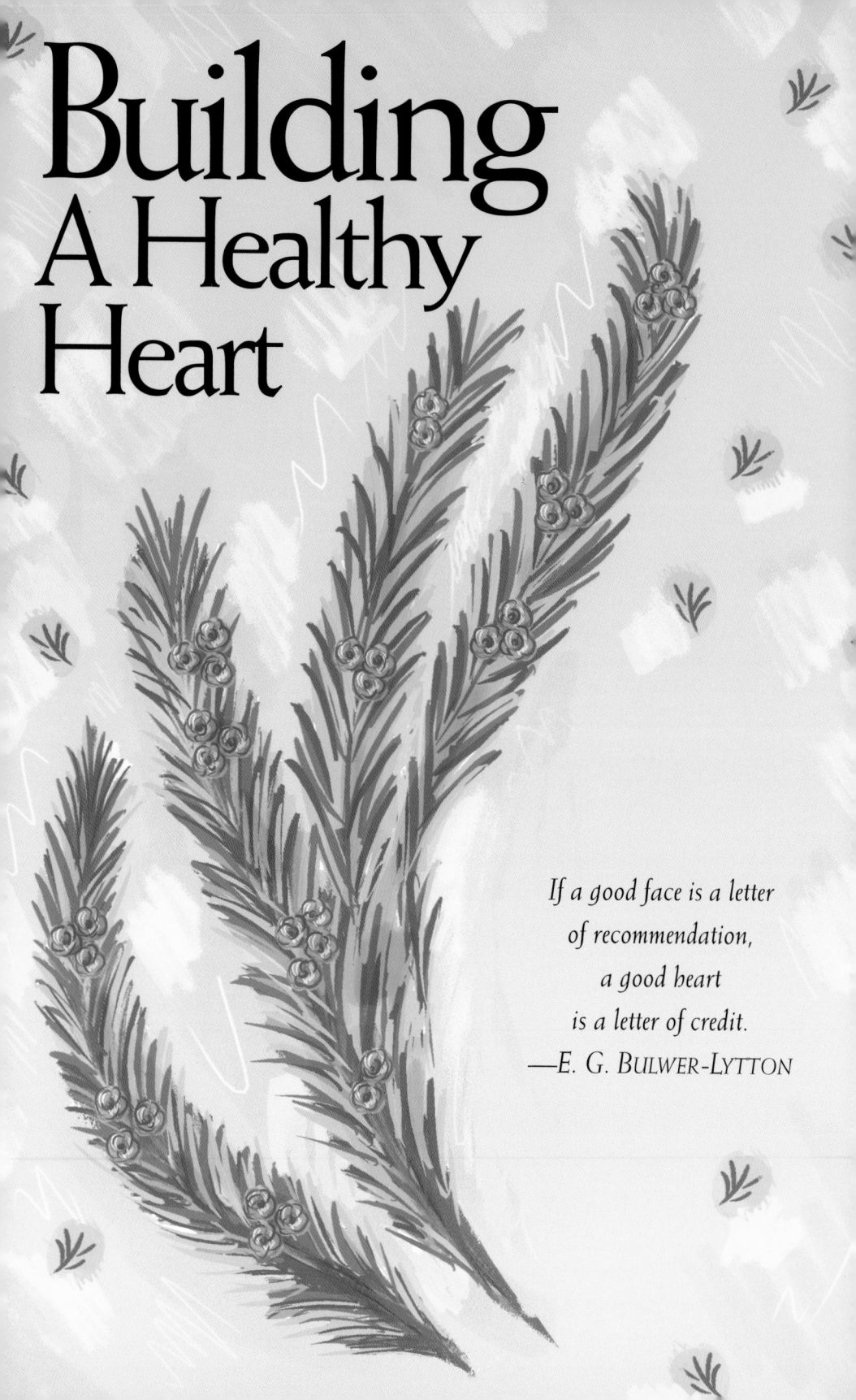

Building
A Healthy
Heart

If a good face is a letter
of recommendation,
a good heart
is a letter of credit.
—E. G. BULWER-LYTTON

THE GOOD HEART

The cardiovascular (circulatory) system is made up of the blood (which carries oxygen, nutrients, wastes, and other substances to and from all parts of the body); the blood vessels (arteries and veins) through which the blood travels; and the heart, a fist-sized muscular organ that pumps the blood into the vessels at the rate of billions of beats in an average lifetime.

When the cardiovascular system is working well, it is a wondrous thing indeed—a high-tech transport and delivery system of essential goods over smooth and traffic-free highways with nary a hitch, miss, or delay. Most of the time we take this fabulous system for granted, until something goes wrong.

To live and let live, without clamor for distinction or recognition; to wait on divine Love; to write truth first on the tablet of one's own heart—this is the sanity and perfection of living, and my human ideal.
—MARY BAKER EDDY

And often something does go wrong. Heart disease is the leading health problem in the Western world.

It is the number one cause of death in the United States, claiming more than 1 million lives a year. In all, an estimated 50 million Americans are afflicted with heart and blood vessel disease.

WHAT IS HEART DISEASE?

The term heart disease covers a number of heart and circulatory problems, including heart conditions caused by birth defects and diseases, conditions such as tachycardia (rapid heartbeat) and arrhythmia (irregular hearbeat), and diseases and malformations of the heart valves and muscles.

But by far the most common form of heart disease—and the focus of this chapter—is coronary artery disease (CAD), also called coronary heart disease. It involves at least one and often all three of the following conditions: atherosclerosis (hardening, narrowing, and blockages of the arteries and to a lesser degree, the veins), high cholesterol levels (hyperlipidemia); and high blood pressure (hypertension).

When the arteries are blocked and become increasingly constricted, the result is poor blood flow, an overworked heart, and sometimes the development of a condition called angina. This is severe chest pain, usually with exertion, that goes away with rest and medication. However, it is almost always a warning that something is amiss with the heart, and in the worst case scenario, angina can be a prelude to a heart attack.

A full discussion of heart disease—and even the place for herbs in its treatment—is beyond the scope of this book. Any heart problem should always be evaluated and monitored by a qualified medical practitioner. Never self-diagnose or self-treat a heart condition. Any treatment for heart disease, herbal or conventional, should be done under the care of your practitioner.

Remember that lifestyle factors are critically important in preventing and managing heart disease: Eat a low-fat diet, get regular aerobic exercise, and don't smoke.

Having said all that, time and scientific research have confirmed that many herbs are beneficial for the heart, and several herbs are specific for treating heart ailments. If you have heart problems, or want to prevent heart disease, talk to your practitioner about using one or more of the herbs

The world stands out on either side—
No wider than the heart is wide;
Above the world is stretched the sky,
No higher than the soul is high.
—EDNA ST. VINCENT MILLAY

that follow as preventive measures or as adjuncts to your conventional medical treatment.

STRENGTHENING YOUR CARDIO-VASCULAR SYSTEM

FIGHTING ATHEROSCLEROSIS WITH HERBS

Herbs that treat the cardiovascular system are called cardiotonics, blood tonics, or alterative tonics. What they all do, over the long term and through one or more specific actions, is help heal and support an overworked or damaged circulatory system. They may do this by detoxifying the blood, promoting good circulation, keeping healthy arteries open and elastic, helping dilate and repair narrowed and damaged arteries, and supporting good kidney and liver function—two organs closely allied with blood circulation.

Each of the herbs that follow can help the heart in many ways. Besides being general heart tonics, they may also lower cholesterol, treat high blood pressure, and help the pain of angina. With your practitioner's approval, they can be taken in combination with many of the other herbs described elsewhere in this chapter.

GARLIC
(Allium sativum)

Truly one of the great herbs, albeit one of the smelliest, garlic has long been revered as a medicinal remedy in both Asian and Western herbal medicine. It has variously been used as an antibiotic and antifungal, and to treat colds, coughs, and digestive disorders.

Today, however, garlic is the subject of considerable study and attention because of its proven role as an adjunct treatment for CAD. Most notably, it reduces both high cholesterol and high blood pressure. It also appears to specifically target and inhibit certain blood conditions that can lead to atherosclerosis. It also helps the kidneys and liver remove toxins from the blood. Allicin, the main ingredient of garlic, together with several other sulfur-containing compounds, are believed responsible for garlic's beneficial effects.

Taken internally for high cholesterol, high blood pressure, and atherosclerosis, garlic is available as cloves and in (odorless and tasteless) tablets. Look for enterically coated tablets.

Caution: Garlic has a blood clot-preventing agent. If you have a blood-clotting disorder, ask your herbalist or doctor about taking garlic.

HAWTHORN
(Crataegus laevigata or
C. oxyacantha)

In recent years, hawthorn has emerged as another of the great heart-healing herbs, with only garlic as a close rival. Its heart-specific therapeutic actions—all rigorously confirmed in many clinical studies—seem legion. It is believed to dilate the blood vessels, thereby facilitating the flow of blood in the arteries and lowering blood pressure. It also appears to increase the pumping force of the heart muscle and to eliminate arrhythmias.

HAWTHORN
(*Crataegus laevigata* or
C. oxyacantha)

Finally, it may have a calming effect on the nervous system (and is even sometimes recommended for insomnia), helping to ease the stress and anxiety that can contribute to an overworked circulatory system.

Hawthorn has been prescribed, along with conventional medical treatments, for high blood pressure, blocked arteries, heart palpitations, angina, and inflammation of the heart muscle. It is available as an extract, dried berries and leaves, and in teas and capsules (by itself or in combination with other herbs).

VITAMIN E—FOOD FOR THE HEART

In two separate studies of over 85,000 women, researchers found that women who ate five ounces or more weekly of nuts (which are high in vitamin E) had 33 percent fewer heart attacks than women who didn't eat nuts. Try sprinkling a handful of nuts over your salad greens every day.

HORSE CHESTNUT
(Aesculus hippocastanum)

There is new and considerable interest in this familiar nut, which can be found strewn across parks, fields, and gardens every fall. Once used as feed for cattle and horses and purportedly to cure horses' coughs, horse chestnut was prescribed by European herbalists in the 1600s as a general tonic and to reduce fevers and treat circulatory problems. On the other side of the Atlantic, Native Americans used the crushed nuts to treat hemorrhoids.

Current interest in horse chestnut centers around its primary chemical constituent, aesculin, which is a known vascular healing agent (it is prescribed for varicose veins) and has been proven to strengthen veins and arteries and inhibit the formation of dangerous blood clots that can lead to heart attack and stroke.

Horse chestnut is available as fresh and dried crushed seed.

Caution: Don't confuse horse chestnut, which is not edible in its natural state, with the sweet chestnut (*Castanea sativa*) of "chestnuts roasting on an open fire" fame. The outer covering of the horse chestnut is toxic; the medicinal part of the seed (nut) is extracted through a careful chemical process. Horse chestnut should be obtained from and prescribed by qualified medical practitioners only.

MOTHERWORT
(Leonurus cardiaca)

The Latin name of this hardy perennial is a tribute to motherwort's long-standing reputation among herbalists as an excellent

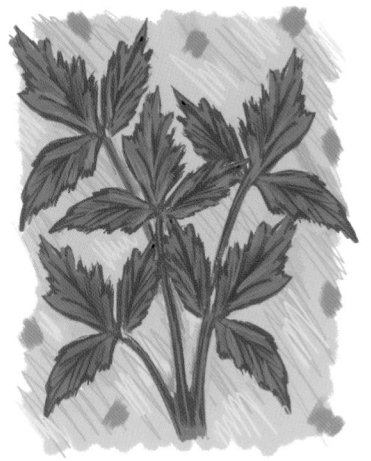

MOTHERWORT
(Leonurus cardiaca)

heart tonic. Research studies confirm that motherwort stabilizes the heart, reduces heart palpitations, treats tachycardia (rapid heartbeat), and eases the pain of angina. It also acts as an antispasmodic and relieves other types of cramping pain. In traditional Chinese medicine, where it is called *yi mu cao*, motherwort is used to treat high blood pressure and edema. (The common name of the plant, motherwort, is a reference to another longtime use of the herb as a treatment for menstrual problems and other women's health conditions; see Chapter 6.)

Taken internally as a heart tonic, motherwort is available in tea, tincture, and capsule forms. It mixes well with hawthorn in combination formulas and teas.

Caution: Motherwort is a uterine stimulant. Do not take it if you suspect you are pregnant or if you are trying to conceive.

LOWERING BLOOD CHOLESTEROL

Cholesterol is a type of fat (or lipid) found naturally in the body and especially in the blood, liver, and brain. The body produces all the cholesterol it needs for certain cellular functions. Problems occur when we add more cholesterol to our bodies through the foods we eat. Too much cholesterol—which binds with proteins in the blood to form lipoproteins—clogs the arteries and increases the risk for athero-sclerosis, heart attack, and stroke. Our bodies' total cholesterol is made up of two kinds of lipoproteins: high-density lipoproteins (HDLs), which are good for the heart, and low-density lipoproteins (LDLs), which are bad for the heart. Several herbs not only reduce total cholesterol levels, but they also raise the levels of good HDLs and lower the bad LDLs. Garlic, as discussed earlier, is one of the great cholesterol-busters. So too are ginger and myrrh.

Lift Up Your Heart in Song!

In the last few years, researchers and laypeople alike have rediscovered the healing benefits of music. Singing is an especially powerful healing experience. Five or ten minutes singing along to a favorite song can chase away the blues and clarify the mind. Singing also expands and strengthens your diaphragm, abdomen, and chest muscles; helps distribute oxygen-rich air and blood to the heart, brain, and other organs; stimulates blood circulation; and aids digestion. Singing also puts a smile on your face, and sometimes that's all the medicine you need.

GINGER
(*Zingiber officinale*)

Ginger is another of the super healing herbs with multiple therapeutic properties (together with a renowned place in the culinary arts!). Both Asian and Western herbalists have traditionally prescribed it for a panoply of ailments: nausea, indigestion, menstrual cramps, motion sickness,

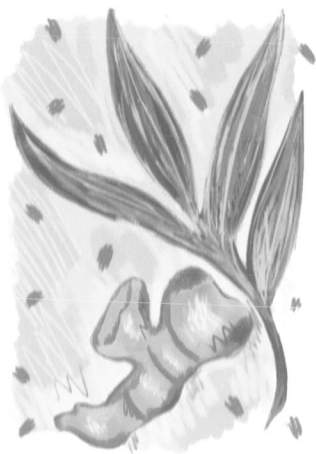

GINGER
(*Zingiber officinale*)

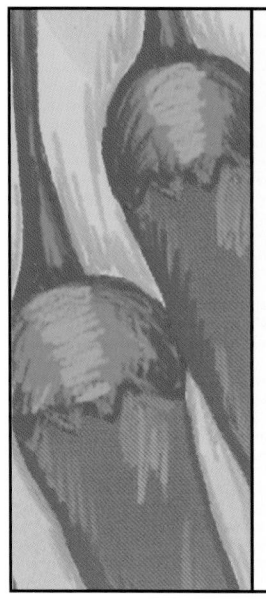

Red Hot

HEART TONIC

Traditional herbalists have long prescribed cayenne (*Capsicum anuum*) as a daily tonic to strengthen the heart, stimulate blood circulation, ease heart palpitations, and prevent heart attacks and strokes. To make a tonic, add 1/4 to 1/2 teaspoon of cayenne (start with the smallest dose you're comfortable with) to 1 cup of juice—tomato juice is the best—and drink up to 3 cups a day.

---

arthritis, colds, and flu. Ginger also is a powerful cholesterol reducer and as good a blood clot-preventing agent as garlic.

Recent research has shown that ginger reduces cholesterol levels by both stimulating the conversion of cholesterol to bile acids and increasing the secretion of the bile. Cholesterol is thus broken down and eliminated more quickly.

Ginger is available as fresh or dried root, powdered root, liquid extract, tablets, capsules, and prepared tea.

To finish the moment, to find the journey's end in every step of the road, to live the greatest number of good hours, is wisdom.

—Ralph Waldo Emerson

Caution: If you have a blood-clotting disorder, ask your herbalist or doctor before taking ginger.

MUKUL MYRRH
(*Commiphora mukul*)

In Chapters 2 and 3 we discussed myrrh's effectiveness in treating cold symptoms and various skin ailments. Myrrh also has an important place among herbs that are used to treat the heart. The myrrh tree is the source of gugulipid, a chemical substance that research studies have shown can significantly reduce both total cholesterol and LDL cholesterol while increasing HDL cholesterol. It also lowers triglyceride levels.

The gugulipid extracted from myrrh is available in 500-milligram capsules that should be taken three times a day as part of a regular regimen for lowering cholesterol. Consult your physician or herbalist about whether gugulipid is right for you, especially if you have kidney disease.

MANAGING HIGH BLOOD PRESSURE

When blood pushes against the walls of the arteries as it travels through the body it creates pressure against the arterial walls. A healthy cardiovascular system promotes a sustained, steady flow of blood, and healthy arteries can take a normal amount of pressure. Normal blood pressure can fluctuate over the course of a day, and can vary from one person to another, from one part of the body to another, or with different physical activities and emotional states. However, high blood pressure (also called hypertension), characterized by chronic, sustained, elevated blood pressure with or without an underlying cause, is one of the constellation of heart problems that is a significant predictor of CAD, heart attack, and stroke.

Blood pressure-lowering herbs (hypotensives) and cardiotonics, such as hawthorn (discussed earlier) and linden and yarrow (described on the following page), work together with a diuretic like dandelion to treat high blood pressure on several levels: by specifically acting to lower blood pressure, by nourishing and strengthening the entire cardiovascular system, and by removing excess fluids from the body and stress on the kidneys.

DANDELION
(Taraxacum officinale)

The lowly dandelion, scourge of those in pursuit of the perfect lawn, has a long and esteemed history of medicinal use, primarily as a diuretic and an alterative herb, although it has many other healing properties. The plant is rich in iron, vitamins A and C (more vitamin A than carrots, in fact) and in the essential nutrient potassium. The latter accounts for its renown as one of the best of the natural diuretics, because it stimulates elimination of excess fluids while supplying the body with potassium. Most diuretics, including the herbal ones, leech potassium from the body.

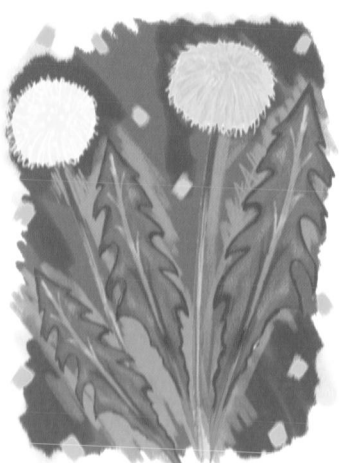

DANDELION
(Taraxacum officinale)

Dandelion's ability to reduce high blood pressure is most directly related to its diuretic properties, but dandelion has other heart-friendly properties that support its blood pressure-reducing action. It detoxifies the blood, nourishes and supports the liver and kidneys (which in turn cleanse the blood), and stimulates the digestive system to break up and eliminate fatty foods.

Dandelion is available in tincture, prepared tea, capsule, and dried or fresh leaves or roots. The fresh leaves may also be eaten in salads.

Caution: If you have heart disease, talk to your practitioner before taking dandelion.

Tilia: The Next Super Herb?

Tilia europea (**linden**) **is only of one of several beneficial species of the** *Tiliaceae* **family.** *Tilia cordata, Tilia platyphyllos,* **and** *Tilia sylvestris* **are also used medicinally. Besides their anxiety-relieving and heart-healing actions,** *Tilia* **blossoms are additionally prescribed for insomnia, panic attacks, incontinence, heavy bleeding, prolapsed uterus, and epilepsy. And laboratory studies suggest that** *Tilia* **also may possess antibacterial, antifungal, anti-inflammatory, and antidiabetic actions!**

LINDEN/LIME BLOSSOMS
(*Tilia europea*)

The beautiful linden flowers or lime blossoms have been used for centuries in traditional herbal teas to treat colds, rheumatic pain, sore throats, and coughs. Linden is also a well-known relaxant and antispasmodic, making it a particularly therapeutic tea where heart problems, so often exacerbated by stress and anxiety, are present.

More recently, linden has been prescribed specifically as a preventive against and treatment for both atherosclerosis and high blood pressure. Its saponin content is similar to that found in horse chestnut (described earlier), and linden appears to have similar therapeutic properties. It acts to dilate constricted veins and arteries and has a healing, tonic effect on damaged blood vessels. It also has diuretic properties that support its blood pressure-lowering effects.

Linden is available as a tincture, dried or fresh chopped flowers, and as prepared tea. It also combines wonderfully with hawthorn and yarrow for a full-spectrum, heart-healing tea.

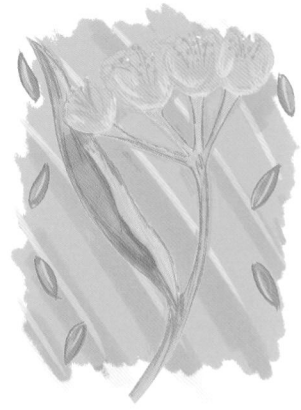

LINDEN/LIME BLOSSOMS
(*Tilia europea*)

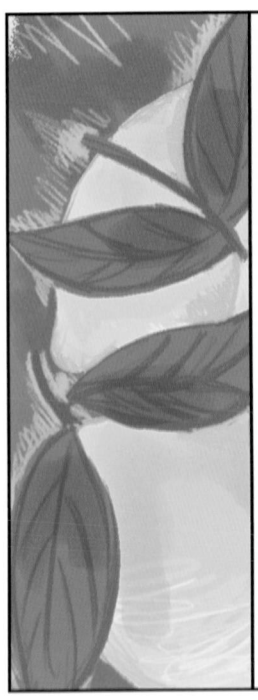

Lemonade

FOR THE HEART

For centuries, Europeans—especially the British—have used the juice made from fresh lemons (*Citrus limon*) to ease heart palpitations associated with stress and anxiety. In fact, lemon has proven stimulating and tonic properties that help to increase blood circulation, nourish the blood, and strengthen overall body functions. To make a heart-toning lemonade, mix the juice of 4 large lemons with 1 quart of spring water and chill slightly. Add the ground rind of one lemon to the lemonade, stir, and sweeten with honey if you like. Drink one or two cups a day.

YARROW
(*Achillea millefolium*)

Since ancient times, yarrow has been known primarily as a great wound healer. In fact, its Latin names comes from the famed Greek warrior, Achilles, who is said to have put yarrow on the bleeding wounds of his soldiers during battle.

Modern research has discovered that yarrow contains multiple therapeutic properties, among them lowering blood pressure, relieving pain, and reducing inflammations. Two major chemical constituents of yarrow, achilletin and achilleine, are believed to prevent blood clotting and help blood coagulate. Another ingredient in yarrow, thujone (which is also found in chamomile), has mild sedating actions. Yarrow also appears to have diuretic properties and it is sometimes used to treat high blood pressure. Yarrow also combines well with hawthorn, linden, cramp bark, and valerian for a powerful cardiotonic and sedating tea.

Yarrow is available as dried herb or tea. Sweeteners can relieve the somewhat bitter taste of yarrow tea.

Caution: Yarrow may produce a rash or diarrhea. If you are allergic to ragweed, you may be allergic to yarrow. If you develop a rash, stop using the herb and consult your doctor.

EASING THE PAIN OF ANGINA

When blood flow to the heart is insufficient or arteries are blocked, a common condition called angina (technically called myocardial ischemia) may occur. Classic angina is characterized by sharp, constricting, and intermittent chest pain that is often preceded by physical exercise or exertion, emotional upset, or exposure to extreme cold. The pain subsides after 5 minutes or so with rest or the use of a medication called nitroglycerin. Another form of angina, which is known as atypical or unstable angina, is pain that occurs at rest. Both forms of angina are signs of heart disease, and unstable angina can be a signal of serious heart trouble.

Treating angina with herbs involves the whole arsenal of heart-healing actions: dilating and repairing damaged, clogged arteries; nourishing and supporting the entire cardiovascular system; facilitating the lowering of high cholesterol and blood pressure; relieving pain; and alleviating anxiety. Just about all the herbs discussed so far have one or more of these properties. Additionally, angelica sinensis and rosemary are especially helpful in treating angina.

ANGELICA SINENSIS/ DONG QUAI
(Angelica sinensis)

Also known as Chinese angelica and *Tang gui*, the sweet-tasting root of angelica sinensis has long been esteemed as one of Chinese herbal medicine's greatest therapeutic herbs, as well as its most potent "fe

male" tonic. Indeed, perhaps no other herb—Western or Asian—is more effective in regulating menstrual cycles and relieving the spasmodic cramps of painful periods (see Chapter 6, "Embracing Good Reproductive Health").

Current research, however, indicates that angelica sinensis may also be a significant treatment for heart disease, especially for arteriosclerosis with accompanying angina. Angelica sinensis appears to increase blood circulation, dilate constricted arteries, relieve constrictive pain, and generally stabilize the heart. All of these properties suggest that angelica sinensis has great potential for treating CAD in general and the symptoms of angina in particular.

Angelica sinensis or dong quai is available in capsule, tincture, extract, and dry bulk forms. In some Asian pharmacies it is available as a tonic called Dong Quai Gin, which can be mixed with tea. Avoid buying root herb that is dry or has a greenish-brown cross-section.

Caution: Before taking this herb, inform your practitioner if you have diarrhea, bloating, heavy menstrual periods, fibroids, or blood-clotting problems.

Wake at dawn with a winged heart and give thanks for another day of loving.
—KAHLIL GIBRAN

ROSEMARY
(Rosmarinus officinalis)

Herbalists believe the leaves of rosemary stimulate the circulatory and nervous systems and have antianxiety properties. The leaves are also believed to contain antispas

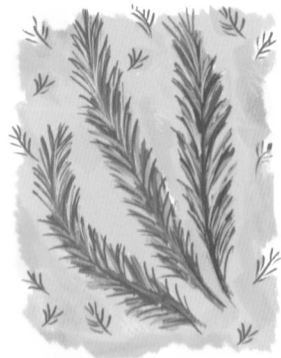

ROSEMARY
(Rosmarinus officinalis)

modic chemicals that relax smooth muscles and relieve pain.

Rosemary's multiple therapeutic actions include tonifying and nourishing the circulatory system, preventing spasms, relieving pain, and alleviating anxiety or stress. All of these therapeutic components are critical aspects of an angina episode, making rosemary a potentially superior herbal remedy for angina in a comprehensive, long-term treatment program.

Rosemary is available as dried herb, tincture, and two types of oil—one for internal use and one for external application (for example, in aromatherapy treatments).

Caution: Do not confuse the rosemary oil meant for internal consumption with the oil for use externally. Never ingest the latter.

Other Helpful Herbs

- **FOR STRENGTHENING AND BALANCING THE HEART:** Asian ginseng, astralagus, barley, blessed thistle, kelp, magnolia, ginkgo

- **FOR REDUCING HIGH BLOOD PRESSURE:** barberry, black cohosh, evening primrose, feverfew, pulsatilla, turmeric

- **FOR IMPROVING CIRCULATION:** cayenne, marigold/calendula, mugwort

- **FOR LOWERING CHOLESTEROL:** flax, pseudoginseng, turmeric

- **FOR ARRHYTHMIAS:** ginkgo

- **FOR ANGINA:** willow

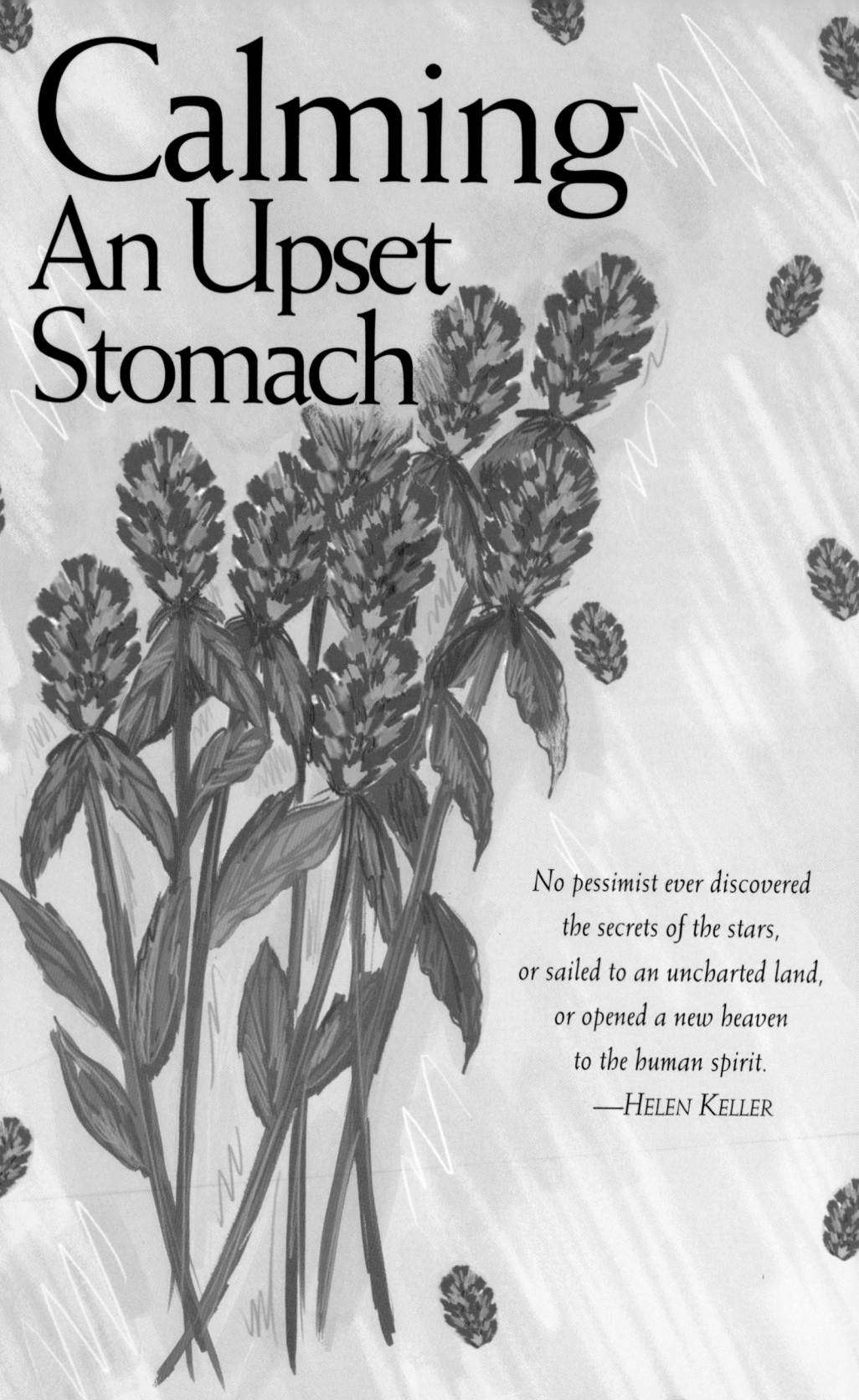

Calming
An Upset
Stomach

No pessimist ever discovered
the secrets of the stars,
or sailed to an uncharted land,
or opened a new heaven
to the human spirit.
—HELEN KELLER

SOOTHING THE GASTROINTESTINAL TRACT

CONSTIPATION

Constipation may present itself as hard stools that are difficult and painful to pass or as the absence of any bowel movement in three days or more. Constipation usually occurs when we don't have enough fiber in our diet, don't exercise, and don't drink enough water. Stress and chronic tension may also bring about this problem. The best way to stay "regular" is to eat a high-fiber diet, drink plenty of water, routinely exercise, and practice some relaxation techniques. Simply heeding the urge to move one's bowels when nature calls (and not later) is also a key factor in avoiding constipation. When necessary, use mild laxatives sparingly to help you get back on schedule.

If you remain constipated despite taking laxatives and especially if you experience pain or abdominal bloating, see a medical practitioner immediately.

CASCARA SAGRADA
(Rhamnus purshiana)

Also known as sacred bark (the Spanish translation of its common name) and California buckthorn, cascara sagrada has commonly been used as a laxative and digestive aid at least since Spanish missionaries (who named the plant) settled in precolonial California. There, western Native Americans had long used a decoction of the tree's bark for its laxative effect.

Today the aged, dried bark of cascara is prized as a gentle, non-habit-forming laxative that can be given to pregnant women, the elderly, and children. Besides its mild laxative properties, cascara also soothes and tones the muscles of the gastrointestinal tract.

Taken internally, cascara may also be prescribed for indigestion and appetite stimulation. Available as dried bark, tincture, and tea, it is sometimes prescribed in combination with carminatives, such as ginger and fennel, to help prevent intestinal cramping.

Caution: Do not take cascara if you suspect you are pregnant or if you are trying to conceive. Do not use for longer than one week at a time. Follow directions for use and do not exceed recommended dosage.

PLANTAIN HERB/PSYLLIUM
(Plantago psyllium, P. ovata)

The seeds of the plantain herb are rich in fiber, making them a safe, bulk-forming laxative that has traditionally been prescribed for constipation and diarrhea. Psyllium, found in many over-the-counter laxatives, such as Metamucil, comes from one of the many plantain plants. (There are more than 200 plantain species.) Because the herb absorbs excess fluid in the intestinal tract and increases stool volume, it can treat both diarrhea and constipation. Plantain herb should not be confused with the plantain banana (Musa acuminata, M. paradisiaca), which has a dried peel that is prescribed for external use in treating warts.

Plantain herb is available as whole seeds, ground or powdered seeds, and in commercial bulk-forming laxative preparations.

Caution: Plantain herb can cause allergic reactions in people who have allergies to dust or grasses. Call your doctor if you have a bothersome allergic reaction. Severe allergic reactions are rare; if you have difficulty breathing, seek emergency help.

To prevent intestinal blockage when taking psyllium as a laxative, you must drink 8 to 10 glasses of water throughout the day. Start using this herb gradually to allow your body to adjust to the increase in fiber. This is good general advice for all laxatives.

Avoid psyllium and other laxatives if you suspect you are pregnant or if you are trying to conceive. Consult your practitioner instead.

DIARRHEA

Frequent, loose, and watery stools, often accompanied by abdominal cramping, herald the onset of diarrhea. Occasional bouts of diarrhea are usually related to viral or bacterial infections, stress, or travel. Chronic diarrhea may be an indication of a more serious gastrointestinal problem, such as a malabsorption disorder in the intestines, Crohn's disease, irritable bowel syndrome, colitis, or diabetes.

Herbs that are mildly astringent, anti-inflammatory, and antispasmodic can all help with diarrhea. Dandelion, featured elsewhere in this book, is a fine antidiarrheal, as are the three herbs featured here.

If diarrhea lasts for more than a few days or is accompanied by excessive pain, cramping, bleeding, fever, or yellow or black stools, see your practitioner immediately.

AMARANTH
(Amaranthus retroflexus)

Amaranth was a staple food of the ancient Aztecs, who endowed it with a mystical connection to the gods and goddesses of fertility, rain, and farming—a connection no doubt made because amaranth grew so readily everywhere and produced abundant crops.

Also known as pigweed and beet-root, amaranth is one of the many *amaranthus* plants that are members of the wild spinach family. Besides being an excellent source of iron, amaranth leaves are also high in vitamin C, beta carotene, potassium, and calcium; the seeds are rich in protein, vitamin E, and the B-complex vitamins. Native Americans used the plant to treat inflammations, toothaches, and bleeding ulcers, but amaranth is also a powerful astringent, and the leaves, made into a tea, are used to treat both indigestion and diarrhea.

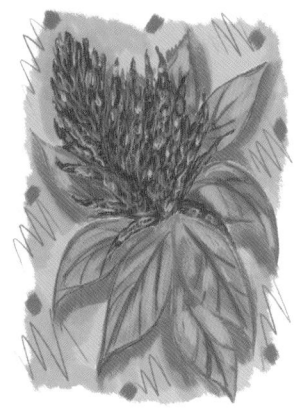

AMARANTH
(Amaranthus retroflexus)

Taken internally for diarrhea and indigestion, amaranth is available as dried leaves, dried seed, and a tea.

BETONY
(Stachys officinalis)

The leaves of the red-purple betony flower were once attributed with magical powers and panacea-like healing properties. Drinking a cup of betony tea at bedtime was believed to ward off nightmares, and chewing the leaves before a party would prevent inebriation. In ancient Rome, betony was believed to cure no fewer than 47 ailments. Also known as bishopswort and wild hop, the dried herb was equally famous in medieval monasteries for curing shortness of breath, but the traditional use of betony, which has analgesic and sedating actions, was in treating "nervous headaches" and anxiety.

Betony has high concentrations of tannin and is one of the bitter astringent herbs that can act as antidiarrheals and digestive aids. Betony is an especially effective treatment for occasional diarrhea brought on by stress. The tea, made from dried leaves and flower tops, has a reputation for being mildly euphoric.

Betony is available as dried herb.

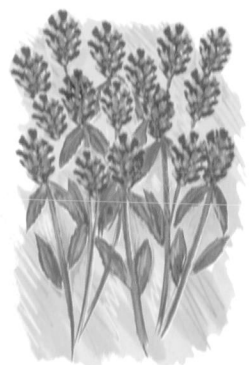

BETONY
(Stachys officinalis)

RED RASPBERRY
(Rubus idaeus)

Red raspberries make for a delicious pie or batch of preserves, culinary uses of the fruit with which we are all familiar. Herbalists, however, value the leaves of the raspberry bush for their high concentrations of tannin, a plant ingredient long used effectively in treating diarrhea and nausea. The raspberry plant has many other medicinal properties, and it is variously prescribed for sore throats, colds, flu, and morning sickness. Recent studies also suggest that red raspberry may reduce levels of glucose (blood sugar) and hence help in the management of diabetes.

Taken internally for diarrhea, nausea, and vomiting, red raspberry is available as dried leaves or berries, tincture, and tea. The tea is made with the dried leaves and makes an especially delicious and healing brew when combined with blackberry (*rubus fruticosus*), another herb that treats diarrhea and soothes the intestinal tract. Many herbalists believe red raspberry tea is most effective against indigestion when it is taken cold.

FLATULENCE AND GAS

Gas, in the form of belching and flatulence, with or without mild gastric pain or discomfort, is a normal part of digestion. Carminative herbs that specifically target gas, indigestion, and colicky pain, are either chewed or drunk in teas to help relieve and even prevent gas. Avoiding foods that typically produce gas for you is the best preventive measure, as is chewing your food well with your mouth closed. (Swallowing air along with your dinner will increase your chances for a bad bout of gas.)

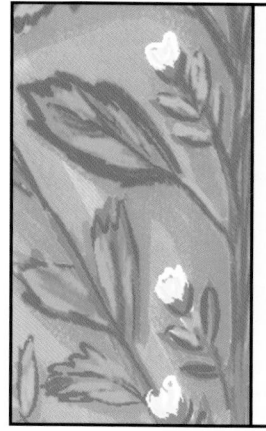

ANISE
(Pimpinella anisum)

Famous for its sharp licorice-like taste and its use as a flavoring in many international cuisines, anise (or aniseed) is one of the oldest and most valued of herbs, used by ancient Egyptians, Greeks, and Arabs. It has always been prized as a uniquely pungent spice used in sweets, curries, and cough preparations, but it is also a powerful herbal remedy for flatulence and cramping indigestion.

The seeds, leaves, and oil of the plant all have therapeutic properties and are commercially available for internal use as teas and chewable seeds. The fresh leaves make a delicious addition to salads.

FENNEL
(Foeniculum vulgare)

Prized for centuries as a food, medicine, and magical charm, fennel is mentioned in the ancient writings of Pliny (who recommended it for improving eyesight) and Hippocrates (who believed it stimulated lactation). During the Middle Ages it was used to chase away demons (the seeds were placed in keyholes to keep evil out of the house) and to treat congestive coughs, a use for which it is still prescribed today. In early America, where the newly arrived Puritans were obliged to fast while attending church services for hours at a time, fennel seeds were chewed to quiet grumbling stomachs (and mask the smell of alcohol on church-goers' breaths!).

Rich in volatile oils that soothe the gastrointestinal tract, fennel is considered a most effective remedy taken internally for flatulence, nausea, and upset stomachs with cramping pain. It can also help curb the appetite and facilitate weight loss. It is available as dried and roasted seeds, fresh and dried leaves, tea, oil, and tincture. The entire plant, and especially the roots and stalks, can be eaten raw or cooked and can be added to any number of dishes.

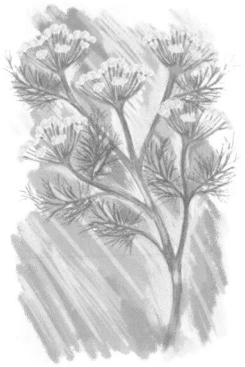

FENNEL
(Foeniculum vulgare)

A CAUTION ABOUT SENNA

The dried pods and leaves of the senna plant (*Cassia angustifolia, C. acutifolia,* and *C. senna*) are used to make a very potent cathartic (laxative). For occasional bouts of severe constipation, senna is an effective laxative in small doses. Recently, however, the herb has reportedly been used in large doses as a purgative for weight-loss and "colonic cleansing" regimens. Regretfully, some deaths have occurred. If you need a laxative, the bulk laxatives, such as psyllium, are a much safer and gentler way to go.

Caution: Do not gather fennel in the wild unless you are an expert at identifying herbs (or have an expert with you). Wild fennel closely resembles the very deadly plant hemlock that grows in the same areas.

I steer my bark with hope in my heart, leaving fear astern.
—THOMAS JEFFERSON

INDIGESTION

Indigestion is an umbrella term covering a host of gastrointestinal upsets that may include one or more of the following: heartburn; flatulence and belching; mild nausea; and especially abdominal pressure, bloating, or cramping pain that can radiate toward the chest. (These symptoms can mimic those of a coronary event; conversely, a heart attack is often first mistaken as indigestion.) Occasional or even daily indigestion that passes in a reasonable time is normal and may be caused by certain foods, overeating, overdrinking, eating too fast or too much, obesity, or smoking. There are effective "stomachic" herbs that promote good digestion and relieve the symptoms of indigestion. The carminative and antispasmodic herbs are also helpful in relieving accompanying gas and cramping.

If indigestion becomes chronic or is accompanied by pain, vomiting, or bleeding, consult your practitioner immediately.

ANGELICA
(*Angelica archangelica*)

Some people today only know angelica as a confectionery used to decorate cakes and as an ingredient in Benedictine. Its medicinal use, however, can be traced back to the early sixteenth century when it was one of several medicines used during the plague. It was frequently prescribed for a host of ailments, including indigestion, flatulence, migraines, and painful menstrual periods. Like other popular herbs of the Middle Ages, angelica was shrouded in mysticism and magic. It was used in wreaths and charms as protection against evil. In addition, two of its common names—St. Michael's Plant and Archangel—are reflections of the fact that it blooms on or near May 8, the feast day of Michael the Archangel (hence its Latin name). Thus it is an "angelic" gift with a spiritually endowed ability to cure anything.

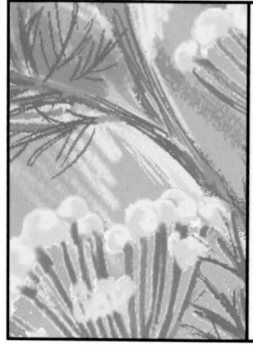

A Stomach-Calming

HOT TODDY

If you don't want to chew anise or fennel seeds, or sip them in teas, they can be combined with warm milk for a pleasant-tasting, stomach-calming, gas-relieving brew. Simmer 1 heaping teaspoon of either anise or fennel seeds in 1 cup of milk for about 10 minutes. Drink hot.

In fact, angelica (which has some of the same properties as angelica sinensis, but to a lesser degree) is a warming tonic and very effective stomachic used internally to treat indigestion, gas, colic, and cramping pain. It also stimulates the appetite. Angelica oil, also called Spirits of Angelica, is sometimes used externally to relieve painful rheumatic joints.

Taken internally as a tea, angelica is prescribed for indigestion, gas, colitis, and cramping abdominal pain. It is available as dried herb (mostly roots) and seeds, oil, tincture, and tea.

Caution: Follow your practitioner's guidelines and only take angelica at prescribed doses. Large doses of the herb can be toxic to the central nervous system. If taken for a long time, angelica can make the skin especially sensitive to sunlight, and appropriate precautions need to be taken.

CARAWAY
(Carum carvi)

Known as a kitchen spice and the ingredient that gives rye bread its distinctive taste, caraway seed is one of the oldest of the healing herbs and has been used medicinally for more than 3,000 years. References to its therapeutic properties were found in an Egyptian scroll at an archeological site that dated back to 1550 B.C.

Caraway's essential oils are high in a substance called carvone, which is specifically effective in treating cramping indigestion accompanied by flatulence. It is also useful in treating colic and some types of menstrual cramping. Caraway has astringent properties as well, and thus can relieve diarrhea.

Caraway is available as fresh and dried seeds, oil, and tea.

PARSLEY
(Petroselinum crispum)

The familiar, feathery leaves of parsley—often used only as a garnish—are a rich source of vitamins C and A, as well as a fine herbal remedy. Parsley has antispasmodic actions and promotes good digestion; it is also a diuretic and a mild laxative. (Eaten raw, parsley is also an excellent breath freshener.)

Parsley is taken internally for indigestion, cramping gastric pain and discomfort, and

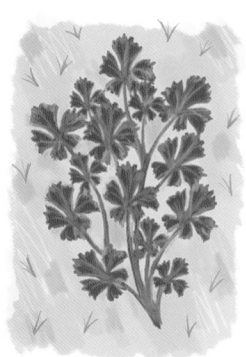

PARSLEY
(Petroselinum crispum)

constipation. It is available as a tincture and as fresh or dried leaves, seeds, stems, and roots.

Caution: If you use this herb frequently as a medicine, you should also eat foods high in potassium, such as bananas, because parsley is also a diuretic, and diuretics deplete the body of potassium.

Parsley has traditionally been used to bring on delayed menstruation. Do not take parsley if you suspect you are pregnant or if you are trying to conceive.

PEPPERMINT
(Mentha piperita)

This common, pleasant-tasting herb has been used as a remedy for indigestion since the time of the pharaohs of ancient Egypt. Menthol, the principal active ingredient, stimulates the stomach lining, reducing the amount of time food spends in the stomach and thereby lessening the chances for indigestion to occur. Peppermint also relaxes the muscles of the digestive system, making it an effective remedy for cramping and colicky pain.

Take peppermint internally for cramps, stomach pain, gas, nausea associated with migraine headaches, travel sickness, insomnia, anxiety, fever, colds, and flu.

Peppermint is available as a commercial tea, tincture, and fresh or dried leaves and flowers.

Caution: Do not ingest pure menthol or pure peppermint; these substances are extremely toxic. Do not take this herb if you suspect you are pregnant or if you are trying to conceive.

IRRITABLE BOWEL

Sometimes called spastic colon or spastic colitis, irritable bowel syndrome (IBS) is the most common—and often most distressing—of digestive ailments, affecting about 15 percent of adults at least once in their lives.

The most obvious symptoms of IBS include diarrhea or frequent loose stools with abdominal pain and cramping, occurring almost always right after meals. Irritable bowel may also involve constipation with abdominal bloating, pain, cramping, and gas, also following meals. An episode of IBS may last several weeks or even months and is often triggered by significant stress or changes in one's life. Herbs that are carminative and stomachic, soothing and anti-inflammatory, and antispasmodic and astringent are all good treatments for IBS. Marshmallow, discussed in Chapter 2, is a very effective remedy. The following herbs also relieve many of the symptoms of an irritable bowel.

HOPS
(Humulus lupulus)

Most famous as an ingredient in brewing beer and ale, hops (or hop, as it is sometimes called) have been used medicinally for centuries as a tonic and a sedative. The female flowers of this climbing vine yield the bitter chemical lupulin, a mild sedative that is widely used to treat insomnia without the morning "headache" and sluggishness that prescription drugs often produce.

Hops also have astringent and antispasmodic properties, which, together with the herb's calming effects, makes it a successful treatment for IBS, colitis, and cramping indigestion, all of which are often related to stress.

Taken internally for digestive complaints, hops are available as dried flowers, tincture, and tea. Fresh hop shoots, also known as hops asparagus, may be chopped and added to salads and vegetables dishes.

Caution: Do not take hops if you have been diagnosed with depression or suspect you are in a depressive state. The sedating and hypnotic actions of hops may exacerbate the depression.

LEMON BALM
(*Melissa officinalis*)

Also commonly known as balm, Melissa, and cure-all, lemon balm is another member of the mint family and one of the gentlest of the calming herbs with potent antispasmodic and antibacterial actions. Besides its wide use for anxiety and insomnia, lemon balm has a reputation among folk herbalists as a universal panacea for gastrointestinal ailments; gallbladder, liver, and heart problems; menstrual and menopausal disturbances; and the symptoms of cold and flu.

Research studies confirm that lemon balm is a potent herbal combination of calmative, carminative, and antispasmodic properties and thus a very effective remedy taken internally for IBS in particular and in-

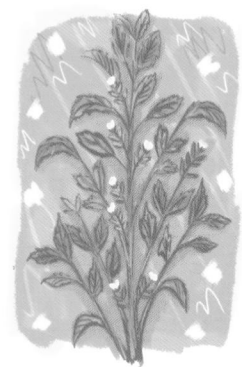

LEMON BALM
(*Melissa officinalis*)

digestion in general—especially when either is accompanied by stress, tension, or anxiety. Lemon balm is available as dried herb, tea, tincture, and oil.

SLIPPERY ELM
(*Ulmus rubra*)

The U.S. Food and Drug Administration calls slippery elm a good demulcent, or soothing agent. Herbalists recommend its external use to ease wounds and skin problems and its internal use for diarrhea and other gastrointestinal disorders. Slippery elm's active ingredient is found in the inner bark, the mucilaginous cells of which expand into a spongy mass when mixed with water.

Its soothing properties make slippery elm a fine remedy for the cramping pain and diarrhea of chronic IBS. It is available in health food stores as capsules, tea, or powder.

Caution: Consult your doctor if you do not improve significantly within two weeks. Some people may be allergic to the powdered bark; if so, discontinue use. Consult your doctor before taking larger-than-recommended doses.

NAUSEA & VOMITING

The nausea and vomiting that sometimes accompany a bout of indigestion are often really the symptoms of gastroenteritis (often called the stomach flu), a general irritation or infection of the gastrointestinal system that can be caused by viruses, bacteria, food poisoning, excessive drinking, or anxiety and stress. Gastritis, an inflammation of the stomach lining, can also cause nausea and vomiting. In Chapter 2 we described several herbs that help treat the nausea and vomiting that accompany colds and flu. Here are two more that are especially soothing for the stomach.

CARDAMOM
(Elettaria cardamomum)

Familiar to most as a delicious kitchen spice, cardamom is a member of the ginger family and has the same "warming" properties of that other famous culinary and medicinal spice. Cardamom is a classic carminative and stomachic herb that can relieve vomiting, indigestion, poor digestion, gas, and diarrhea; as an antispasmodic, it also eases the stomach and intestinal cramping that might accompany all those ailments. Additionally, cardamom has proved an especially useful stomach and digestive treatment when there is general weakness and debilitation.

Taken internally for vomiting, nausea, indigestion, gas, diarrhea, and cramping, cardamom is available as ground seeds, powder, and tea.

OSWEGO TEA/BEE BALM/RED BERGAMOT
(Monarda didyma)

The brilliant red flowers and richly aromatic citrus scent of Oswego tea has made this member of the horsemint family a prized ornamental flower for centuries, although it grows wild in many of North America's damp woodlands. It became a popular tea in the late 1700s when it replaced Indian tea after the infamous Boston Tea Party. It was variously named Oswego tea (for the Oswego Indians who shared it with early settlers), bee balm (for its special attraction to those insects), and red bergamot (for its orange scent, so reminiscent of bergamot orange, a European mint plant).

Rich in thymol (an antibacterial and antifungal) and tannins (which traditionally treat such ailments as diarrhea, ulcers, and colitis), Oswego tea is taken internally to relieve vomiting, nausea, and flatulence. It is available as dried or fresh leaves and flowers, tea, and oil.

More
Helpful Advice
BECOME LIKE CHILDREN AGAIN . . .

Practitioners of East Indian Ayurvedic medicine believe that chronically poor digestion is the root cause of most illness. It isn't surprising then that yoga, India's ancient and now very popular practice of physical exercises, contains many yogic postures (body movements and positions) that promote proper digestion and relieve gas and indigestion. One of the simplest of yoga postures for indigestion relief is the Child pose: Kneel on a carpeted floor, then sit back on your heels, knees together. Slowly start bending forward from your hips, letting your arms gently drop to the floor alongside your knees, with palms up. Keep bending forward until your upper body is resting on your knees and your forehead is just touching the floor. Take long, deep breaths through your nose and stay in this position for at least 30 seconds. Slowly sit up and take a deep breath. Not only will your tummy feel better, you'll feel relaxed and refreshed.

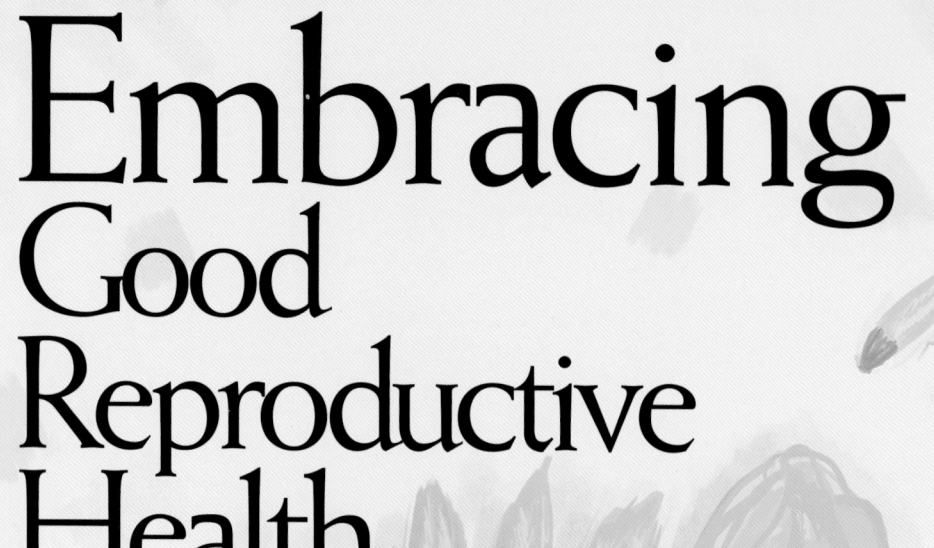

Embracing
Good
Reproductive
Health

Dream lofty dreams,
and as you dream,
so shall you become.
Your vision is the promise
of what you shall
at last unveil.
—JOHN RUSKIN

MENOPAUSE

Menopause is technically defined as the end of menstrual periods, but it is in fact much more: a collection of symptoms that may begin as early as 40 (when the symptoms are called perimenopausal) and continue for 10 or more years while levels of the hormones estrogen and progesterone drop dramatically.

Hot flashes, irregular periods, muscle aches and pains, excessive sweating, disturbed sleep, mood swings, forgetfulness, tender breasts, and abdominal bloating are common physical symptoms of the low hormone levels that characterize menopause. So too are dry skin and nails, brittle and thinning hair, and vaginal dryness and irritation. Any one of those symptoms can upset a woman's physical, mental, and emotional well-being.

A host of herbs are available to treat menopausal symptoms. For physical symptoms, there are healing herbs with diuretic, analgesic, anti-inflammatory, immune-boosting, and vasorelaxing actions, all of which can relieve abdominal bloating, muscle aches and pains, breast tenderness and swelling, general fatigue, dry skin and hair, and the hot flashes caused by constricting blood vessels. For emotional symptoms, there are sedating, mood-elevating, and sleep-inducing herbs.

Here we highlight three of the best herbs for treating the physical and emotional symptoms of perimenopause and menopause: angelica sinensis, black cohosh, and Asian ginseng. Chaste tree and wild yam are two other fine herbal remedies for these symptoms. We feature both herbs later in this chapter in the sections on PMS and menstrual problems.

ANGELICA SINENSIS/DONG QUAI
(Angelica sinensis)

Also known as Chinese angelica root and *tang gui*, angelica sinensis is considered the premier "female" herb in Asia, used by millions of women every day to regulate hormone function, tonify (strengthen) the reproductive organs, and promote healthy blood circulation. Modern research into the herb's tonifying properties confirms that angelica lowers blood pressure, slows the pulse rate, relaxes the heart muscle, and stabilizes blood sugar levels. It also has sedating and calming effects, and can improve the appearance of skin and hair. It also helps in the absorption and utilization of vitamin E, which is essential to good circulation and a healthy heart.

Angelica sinensis's "tonifying" effects are especially useful in treating the fatigue and general feeling of debilitation that often accompany menopause, due in part to constricting arteries (caused by low estrogen levels), poor blood circulation, and intermittent bouts with insomnia.

Taken internally for the symptoms of menopause and as a female tonic, angelica sinensis is available as dried herb, tea, tincture, and capsules.

Caution: Do not use this herb if you have diarrhea or abdominal bloating. Consult your medical practitioner instead.

BLACK COHOSH
(Cimicifuga racemosa)

What angelica sinensis is to the East, black cohosh is to the West. This yellow-flowered member of the buttercup family, one of the great native herbs of America, has been variously known through the centuries as bugbane (for its effectiveness in repelling bugs; cimicifuga is Latin for bug repellant), snakeroot, and yellow ginseng. Native Americans used black cohosh for a variety of "female" ailments, and early American colonists used it to treat everything from yellow fever to nervous disorders and snakebites. Modern herbalists still use black cohosh tea to soothe a sore throat.

However, it is the plant's estrogen-like components (technically called phytoestrogens), particularly its chemical constituents actein and triterpene, that have made black cohosh one of the most effective herbal treatments for many of the symptoms of menopause. In Europe black cohosh has been the subject of serious research for more than 50 years. In Germany it is the most widely prescribed (and used) natural alternative to conventional estrogen replacement therapy.

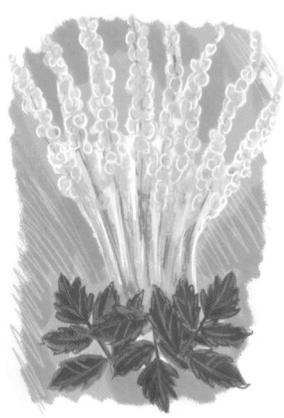

BLACK COHOSH
(Cimicifuga racemosa)

Black cohosh is taken internally to relieve hot flashes, depression, night sweats, anxiety, heart palpitations, and vaginal dryness. It is available as dried herb, tea, tincture, and capsules.

Caution: Use black cohosh only under the supervision of a medical practitioner. Overdoses or prolonged use can cause dizziness, diarrhea, vomiting, abdominal pain, joint pains, and lowered heart rate. If any of these symptoms develop while you are taking black cohosh, stop using it and call your practitioner immediately. There is also some indication that inappropriate use of black cohosh may contribute to abnormal blood clotting, liver problems, and breast tumors.

To exist is to change, to change is to mature, to mature is to go on creating oneself endlessly.
—*HENRI BERGSON*

ASIAN GINSENG
(*Panax ginseng*)

Growing on the mountains of northeast China, Asian ginseng—or Panax ginseng—is the most potent form of ginseng and the greatest of all the "tonic" herbs, celebrated in herbal history for thousands of years. With its yellow-green flowers and red berries, it looks like American ginseng (*Panax quinquefolius*), but the stalk is longer. Other related ginseng species, including Siberian ginseng (*Eleutherococcus senticosus*), Himalayan ginseng (*Panax pseudoginseng*), and Japanese ginseng (*Panax japonicum*), all have unique healing properties, but none is as potent and medically esteemed as Asian ginseng.

Considerable clinical research confirms that the herb significantly reduces the mental and physical fatigue characteristic of menopause, increases mental clarity, generally strengthens the body's overall functioning, and helps alleviate the damage caused by physical and emotional stress. All of these healing properties make Asian ginseng a superb herbal supplement during menopause.

Taken internally for fatigue, stress, strengthening of the immune system, and regulation of hormone levels, Asian ginseng is available as dried herb and tincture, and in a variety of commercial preparations, including capsules and tea.

Caution: Use ginseng only under the care of a medical practitioner. Side effects are usually minimal and may include headaches, insomnia, breast soreness, or skin rashes. In some susceptible individuals, however, Asian ginseng may precipitate asthma attacks, increased blood pressure, heart palpitations, or uterine bleeding. If these symptoms occur, consult your practitioner immediately.

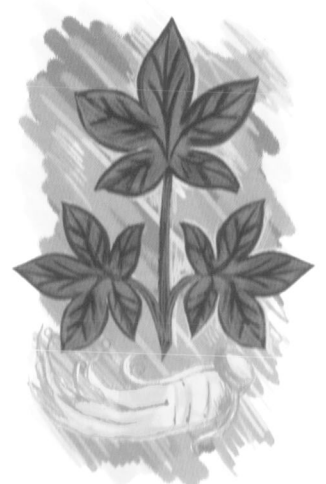

A S I A N   G I N S E N G
(*Panax ginseng*)

> *Grow up as soon as you can.*
> *It pays. The only time you really*
> *live fully is from thirty to sixty. . .*
> *The young are slaves to dreams;*
> *the old servants of regrets.*
> *Only the middle-aged have all*
> *their five senses. . .*
> —WILLIAM HERVEY ALLEN

MENSTRUAL PROBLEMS

Menstrual problems may start with the first menstrual period and continue through menopause. The most common menstrual problems are painful cramps (dysmenorrhea); heavy or excessively long periods (menorrhagia); and scanty, irregular, or delayed periods (amenorrhea). These problems may be chronic or occur only occasionally, and the duration and intensity of any one of these conditions will vary greatly from individual to individual.

Any menstrual problem that continues for more than one cycle should always be evaluated by a qualified medical practitioner. After that, you will find many herbal remedies available for each of the three common menstrual problems. Because several herbs are useful for treating more than one ailment, it is useful to read through the entire section. Finally, sedating and calming herbs, such as chamomile, kava kava, and valerian, are also useful for treating menstrual problems and PMS. These herbs are discussed in detail in Chapter 8.

HERBS FOR PAINFUL CRAMPS

CRAMP BARK
(Viburnum opulus)

In popular use in America since the early 1800s—and long before that by Native Americans—cramp bark has sedating and antispasmodic actions and is a general uterine tonic. It is one of the most effective herbs for treating menstrual cramping and pain, including lower back pain. The main ingredients in cramp bark—viburnin, a powerful antispasmodic, and valerianic acid, the same potent sedative found in valerian and hops—are responsible for the herb's effectiveness in treating cramping pain. Cramp bark, also an anti-inflammatory, relaxes muscles, reduces pain and swelling, and exerts a gentle sedating effect. Also known as Guelder rose and cranberry tree (its fruit resembles real cranberries, but they are toxic if eaten raw), cramp bark was used by Native Americans as a tonic for strengthening and normalizing the uterus after childbirth.

Cramp bark is available as dried herb, capsules, or tincture.

Caution: The fresh berries are toxic.

FALSE UNICORN ROOT
(Chamaelirium luteum)

Considered one of the finest tonics for the female reproductive system, false unicorn root—also known as fairywand, devil's-bit, and helonias—was a staple of Native American medicine, used for centuries to treat women's ailments. Its popularity spread to early settlers who also used it for headaches, colic, and depression.

The powdered root is most widely used today for regulating menstrual periods and relieving menstrual pain and cramping. It is a stimulating tonic with antispasmodic action. Taken internally for irregular and painful periods and for treating infertility and impotence, false unicorn root is a slow-acting herbal remedy, usually given over the course of several months. It is often combined in herbal teas and formulas with

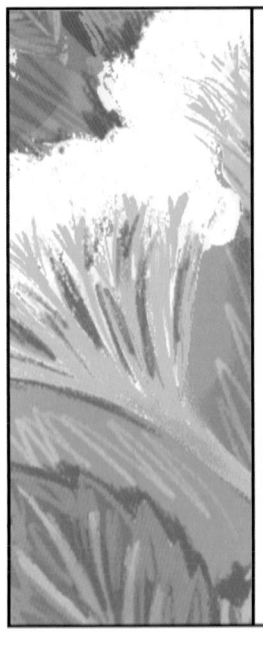

Soothing

HERBAL BATH

For a healing herbal bath that relieves aching muscles, calms frazzled nerves, and promotes a restful night's sleep, mix together in a small bowl 1 teaspoon dried herb each of chamomile, hops, lemon balm, St. John's wort, valerian, and wild yam. Place mixture in a piece of cheesecloth or muslin and secure well with string. (Many herb and natural food stores sell small muslin drawstring bags just for this purpose.) Place herbal mixture in tub and allow hot water to run over it as tub fills. Soak in bath for at least 20 minutes.

cramp bark, and it is available as dried herb, tincture, and capsules.

Caution: Because of its uterine-stimulating action, do not take false unicorn root if you suspect you are pregnant or if you are trying to conceive.

WILD YAM
(Dioscorea villosa)

Popular during the eighteenth and nineteenth centuries as a remedy for menstrual pain, wild yam is currently enjoying a popular comeback. Wild yam extract, taken from the root, contains an alkaloid substance that relaxes the abdominal muscles. Consequently, it is often prescribed to relieve menstrual cramping and pain. Herbalists also prescribe wild yam (and many menopausal women self-treat with it) for its alleged estrogen- and progesterone-like properties and thus its purported ability to relieve some of the symptoms of perimenopause and menopause, especially hot flashes and irregular, heavy periods. For this

purpose, wild yam is often used in creams and applied topically. Medical practitioners debate the effectiveness of this treatment, although many women report considerable success using wild yam for this purpose.

Wild yam is available as dried root, tincture, capsules or creams.

Caution: Consult a practitioner before using wild yam as a progesterone supplement.

HERBS FOR HEAVY OR PROLONGED MENSTRUAL PERIODS

LADY'S MANTLE
(Alchemilla vulgaris, A. xanthochlora)

Once revered by medieval alchemists (hence its genus name *Alchemilla*), who believed the dew of the plant was essential to

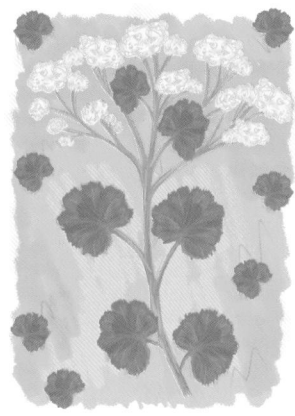

LADY'S MANTLE
(Alchemilla vulgaris,
A. xanthochlora)

the process of changing ordinary metals into gold or silver, lady's mantle became popular for its real therapeutic actions: relieving heavy menstrual bleeding and helping ease menstrual cramping and pain. Also known as breakstone, lady's mantle is an effective diuretic and astringent that has been used to treat gallstones. It also has sedating and sleep-promoting properties and is frequently combined with slippery elm to soothe and relax tense abdominal muscles.

Taken internally for excessive menstrual bleeding and cramping pain, lady's mantle is available as dried herb, tea, and tinctures.

Caution: Do not take lady's mantle if you suspect you are pregnant or if you are trying to conceive.

SHEPHERD'S PURSE
(Capsella bursa-pastoris)

Also known as shepherd's heart, shepherd's purse got its common and Latin names centuries ago because the flat seed pouches of the plant resembled the purses that shepherds used to wear on their belts. (The Latin *capsella* means "purse" or "pocket.")

Today, shepherd's purse is considered one of the most effective herbal remedies for stopping any kind of bleeding. It is frequently prescribed for heavy menstrual bleeding, particularly that associated with perimenopause and menopause. The herb is also helpful in regulating menstrual cycles. Shepherd's purse has astringent and diuretic properties and acts as a general alterative tonic. Research additionally suggests that it may help support the pituitary gland and regulate progesterone levels.

Shepherd's purse is available as dried herb, tea, tincture, and capsules.

HERBS FOR SCANTY, IRREGULAR, OR DELAYED MENSTRUAL PERIODS

BLUE COHOSH
(Caulophyllum thalictroides)

A well-known uterine tonic and stimulant, blue cohosh has been used effectively to tonify and stimulate a sluggish uterus and to help promote menstrual flow. The medicinal root of the plant first garnered attention for its use by Native American women (it is sometimes called squaw root, as are many other native herbs) who drank a tea made from the root for two weeks prior to giving birth, resulting in mostly pain-free deliveries.

Blue cohosh has both a stimulating and a strong antispasmodic effect on voluntary and involuntary muscles, especially those of the uterus. It is most frequently prescribed to bring on delayed menstrual periods and normalize irregular periods with either scanty or heavy bleeding. The dried root also has astringent properties that are responsible for its effectiveness in treating heavy bleeding.

Blue cohosh is available as dried herb, tincture, tea, and capsules.

Caution: Avoid the seeds of the blue cohosh plant; they are poisonous. Blue cohosh is an emmenagogue; that is, an herb used specifically to promote menstruation. Do not take it if you suspect you are pregnant or if you are trying to conceive.

MUGWORT LEAF
(Artemisia argyi, A. vulgaris)

Mugwort leaf is prescribed by Asian and Western herbal practitioners for a variety of gynecological problems. In the West it is also prescribed for digestive complaints and for depression. It is most frequently used, however, as a uterine tonic specifically for treating menstrual problems, including delayed or scanty periods. Mugwort also has antispasmodic and sedating properties, making it useful for relieving painful menstrual cramping and promoting general relaxation.

Taken internally, mugwort is also sometimes prescribed for heavy bleeding. It is often combined with ginger in herbal teas and formulas to relieve menstrual pain. Mugwort is available as dried herb, tincture, tea, and capsules.

Caution: Mugwort is an emmenagogue; that is, an herb used specifically to promote menstruation. Do not take it if you suspect you are pregnant or if you are trying to conceive.

PENNYROYAL
(Mentha pulegium)

Pennyroyal—an especially pungent member of the mint family also known as English pennywort and pudding grass— is the strongest of the uterine tonics and menstrual

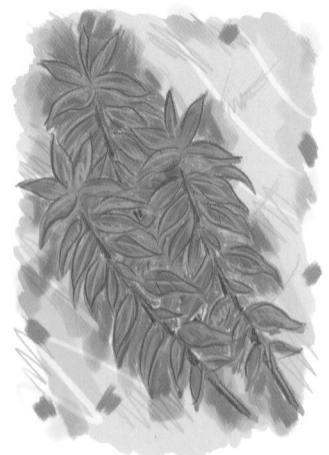

PENNYROYAL
(Mentha pulegium)

regulators we discuss here. Long used as a medicinal herb, it was equally famous as a very effective insect repellant, especially noxious to fleas and mosquitoes. (Pulegium is a derivation of the Latin *pulex*, meaning flea.)

Pennyroyal's major chemical ingredient is pulegone, which is believed responsible for most of the herb's therapeutic actions. It is most frequently prescribed for irregular or scanty menstrual periods and for delayed menstruation. It is also a stimulating uterine tonic. Pennyroyal may additionally be used to treat flatulence, headache, and nausea.

Taken internally, pennyroyal is available as dried herb, tea, tincture, and capsules.

Caution: Take pennyroyal only under the care of a qualified practitioner, as appropriate and precise dosing is critical when using this herb. Do not take it if you have kidney disease or if you suspect you are pregnant or are trying to conceive. Once erroneously labeled a common abortifacient (in fact, the dose needed for an aborting effect is highly toxic), pennyroyal nevertheless is a strong emmenagogue and uterine stimulant.

OSTEOPOROSIS

Osteoporosis is a chronic condition in which the bones gradually thin and weaken, greatly increasing the chance of bone fractures—a situation that is exacerbated by age and can cause disability and death. Women are especially susceptible to osteoporosis because they have thinner, lighter bones, and because there appears to be a link between the hormonal changes of menopause and an accelerated weakening of the bones. Prevention is the greatest weapon against osteoporosis, because once it has begun it is difficult to reverse. Two primary preventive measures are eating nutritious foods rich in calcium and other minerals and doing regular weight-bearing exercises.

Several herbs that are rich in minerals and other nutritious substances may offer supplemental help in an osteoporosis prevention program. Here are two of the most frequently prescribed, mineral-rich herbs.

HORSETAIL
(Equisetum arvense)

Horsetail has been valued since ancient times for its ability to bind and heal connective tissue. It is rich in silica, which helps mend broken bones and form collagen, a constituent of bones and tissues. The latter action makes horsetail an excellent choice as a supplemental herb for possible prevention of osteoporosis. Horsetail is also effective in stopping bleeding and increasing urine production. It is often prescribed for the pain of rheumatism and arthritis, wounds, urinary ailments, and benign prostate disorders.

Taken internally for strengthening bones, for broken bones or sprains, and for joint pain, horsetail is available as dried or fresh herb, capsules, and tincture.

Caution: Take horsetail only under the care of a qualified practitioner and only in minimal doses. Extended use may cause kidney or heart damage. Take with caution if you have kidney or heart disease. Minor side effects may include upset stomach, diarrhea, or increased urination. Serious side effects can include kidney or lower back pain, pain on urination, or cardiac problems. If you experience any of these symptoms, discontinue use and contact your practitioner immediately.

COMMON OAT/ OAT STRAW
(Avena sativa)

Oats were once a cherished herbal remedy—and food—used by herbalists and rural medical practitioners for centuries. They were prized as a sedative and a treatment for a variety of medical problems, including depression, constipation, insomnia, and general debilitation from illness and poor nutrition. Always a staple food product worldwide, oats nevertheless fell out of favor as an herbal medicine for many years. Today many people know it mostly as a cereal and the main ingredient in Aveeno—

after its Latin name *avena*, which means "nourishing"—a popular commercial bath product used to soothe rashes, poison ivy, and dry skin.

Oats are making a comeback as an herbal remedy and supplement, however, due in great part to the fact that oat is indeed one of the most nourishing of the herbal plants. It is rich in proteins; vitamin E, vitamin K, and the B vitamins; and phosphorus, iron, zinc, manganese, and potassium. Its sedating effect is due to avenine, one of the plant's chemical ingredients. It is one of the best of the high-mineral-content herbs that may be useful in preventing osteoporosis.

Taken internally for its nutritive and sedating properties, oats may be eaten as cereal, porridge, and in baked goods. Oats are also available as grains and kernels.

PREMENSTRUAL SYNDROME

Premenstrual syndrome (PMS) is difficult to define. The type and intensity of symptoms vary greatly from woman to woman, and well over 100 possible PMS symptoms have been identified. Generally, PMS is experienced as 7 to 14 days of significant physical, psychological, and emotional discomfort, the degree of which may range from simply annoying to intensely disruptive. Largely caused by hormonal swings and individual chemistry and lifestyle, some of the symptoms of PMS include bloating

and weight gain; breast pain and swelling; acne or herpes outbreaks; headaches, backaches, and joint pain; constipation or diarrhea; anxiety, irritability, or depression; fatigue; and nausea. The herbs featured here are proven remedies for PMS. They combine diuretic, anti-inflammatory, hormone-regulating, and pain-relieving properties. As with menstrual problems, many of the sedating and calming herbs featured in Chapter 8 are also helpful in treating PMS.

CHASTE TREE
(*Vitex agnus-castus*)

Sometimes called chasteberry or monk's pepper, the flowers of the chaste tree plant were believed to lower the libido, and the

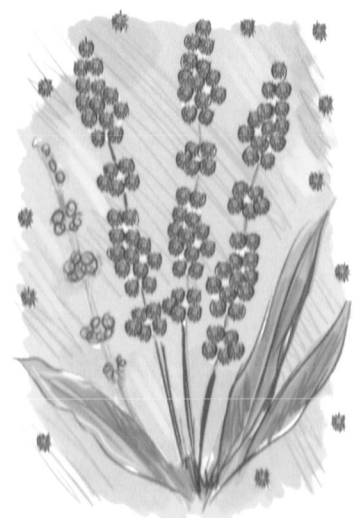

CHASTE TREE
(*Vitex agnus-castus*)

herb derived its name in part from the medieval notion that placing the plant near a young monk's vestments would help him keep his vow of chastity.

Since ancient times, herbalists have used the fruit of the chaste tree to regulate the menstrual cycle, a use for which it is considered one of the finest herbs available. Today it is most frequently prescribed for PMS, for which it is considered by many to be the best herbal remedy. Taken internally, chaste tree can relieve the tension, anxiety, mood swings, bloating, and disturbed sleep that characterize PMS.

Chaste tree also contains progesterone-like chemicals that make it a superior treatment for the irregular and heavy menstrual periods that often signal the perimenopausal years. Clinical trials have confirmed that chaste tree regulates the ratio of estrogen to progesterone and thus can normalize menstrual cycles (by increasing the time between periods) and decrease heavy bleeding (by shortening the length of the menstrual periods themselves). Extracts of the dried berries—in capsule or tincture form—also have proved effective in treating the mild depression associated with menopause.

Taken internally for PMS, menstrual problems, and menopausal symptoms, chaste tree is available as dried herb, capsules, extract, and tincture.

EVENING PRIMROSE
(Oenothera biennis)

Evening primrose, so named because its large, yellow flowers open in the evening, is a perennial plant native to North America. The fresh leaves and stems have been variously used internally to treat gastritis, colds, whooping cough, cramps, and asthma. Externally, evening primrose helps heal wounds and certain skin conditions. Also known as evening star, the herb has been increasingly prescribed for PMS. It is a mild

astringent with sedating and antispasmodic properties, good for treating the bloating, tension, pain, and anxiety that frequently characterize the premenstrual period.

Most recently, research and popular attention has focused on the additional therapeutic actions of evening primrose oil, which is extracted from the seeds. One of the oil's primary actions is relieving the breast pain and sensitivity that many premenstrual women experience. Repeated studies show that evening primrose oil contains an essential fatty acid, gammalinolenic acid (GLA), that is converted in the body to hormone-like substances (prostaglandins) that regulate many body functions and reduce inflammation and pain. This is especially significant in the treatment of PMS, as the same studies have shown that women who experience PMS with breast pain have very low concentrations of GLA. Evening primrose oil also appears to have potent anti-clotting properties, making it a potential treatment for heart attack prevention.

Taken internally, evening primrose may also be prescribed for certain skin conditions, such as eczema, and for arthritis. It is available as dried herb (leaves), oil, and capsules.

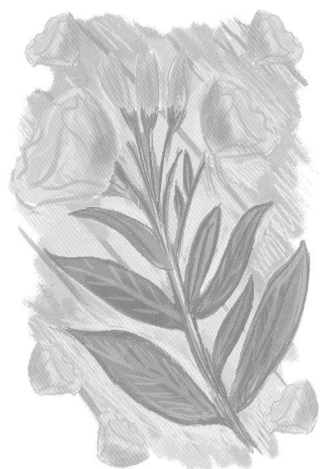

EVENING PRIMROSE
(Oenothera biennis)

Caution: Do not confuse evening primrose with English primrose, a similar-looking but very poisonous plant. If you have a blood-clotting disorder, consult your practitioner before taking evening primrose oil. Do not take evening primrose if you suspect you are pregnant, or if you are trying to conceive.

UVA-URSI
(Arctostaphylos uva-ursi)

Uva-ursi is another of the fine diuretic and astringent herbs that are particularly helpful in relieving premenstrual bloating by promoting urine production and elimination. Prescribed by herbalists for a number of urinary tract infections, including cystitis and prostatitis, uva-ursi is also used to treat minor wounds and to shrink and tone the uterus after childbirth. Its leaves contain arbutin, which is converted in the urinary tract to the infection-fighting antiseptic hydroquinone. Like other diuretics, it is also useful in the treatment of high blood pressure. Its value in treating PMS lies in its diuretic and antiseptic properties.

Taken internally, uva-ursi is available as dried herb, tincture, and tea (alone or in combination with other ingredients, such as marshmallow).

Caution: Taking uva-ursi may produce dark green urine; this is harmless. Because diuretics leech potassium from the body, remember to eat potassium-rich foods, such as bananas, while taking the herb. At the same time, avoid acidic foods and vitamin C, because uva-ursi works only in an alkaline environment.

Take uva-ursi only on the advice of your medical practitioner in the smallest prescribed doses. High doses can cause stomach upset, tinnitus (ringing in the ears), nausea, and convulsions. If any of these symptoms occur, contact your practitioner immediately. Do not take uva-ursi if you

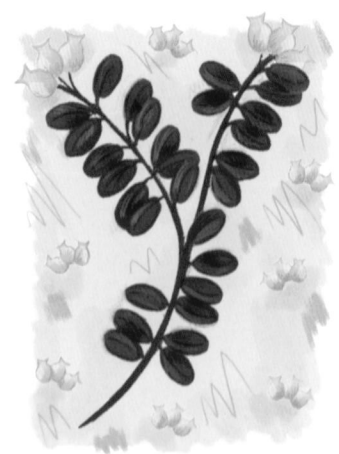

U VA - U R S I
(Arctostaphylos uva-ursi)

suspect you are pregnant or if you are trying to conceive.

THE PROSTATE AND BENIGN PROSTATIC HYPERPLASIA

The walnut-size prostate gland that surrounds the male urethra (the tube that transports urine for elimination) is responsible for manufacturing seminal fluid to carry sperm and regulating the flow of urine from the bladder. The prostate enlarges as a natural byproduct of the aging process and male hormonal changes. An enlarged prostate, putting pressure on the urethra, may cause both urinary and sexual problems.

The most common form of prostate enlargement is called benign prostatic hyperplasia (BPH), which is characterized by increased frequency of urination (with or without burning or pain), reduced force and amount of urine, urgent and frequent nighttime urination, and difficulty emptying the bladder. An enlarged prostate may also be the result of a urinary tract or bladder infection; prostatitis and urethritis are common infections with many of the same symptoms of BPH, plus fever and pain.

Prostate problems must always be evaluated by a qualified practitioner. Infections will require antibiotics, and many of the symptoms of BPH mimic the symptoms of prostate cancer. Careful medical assessment is crucial. Once a diagnosis has been made, the

Zap it! With Zinc & Tomatoes

Research suggests that zinc is important to maintaining prostate health. Add some zinc-rich foods to your diet, including sunflower seeds, wheat bran, oatmeal, oysters, and pumpkin seeds. And throw in two to three servings of tomatoes a week while you're at it. Another study has demonstrated that lycopenes, substances found in tomatoes, may reduce the risk of prostate cancer.

herbs featured here are particularly effective in helping treat BPH and urinary tract infections. Take these herbs only under the advice of your practitioner.

PYGEUM
(Pygeum africanum)

Pygeum is a native herb of southern Africa that is now found throughout North America. The bark of this evergreen tree has long been used in Africa and America to treat a variety of male urinary tract disorders, such as prostatitis (inflammation of the prostate) and urethritis (inflammation of the urethra). Recent research suggests that pygeum may additionally help alleviate many of the symptoms of BPH, including decreased urine flow, reduced force of urine flow, and enlarged prostate. It may also be useful in helping treat prostate cancer.

Taken internally, pygeum is available as dried bark and tea.

Do I contradict myself?
Very well then, I contradict myself
(I am large, I contain multitudes).
—WALT WHITMAN

SAW PALMETTO
(Serenoa repens, S. serrulata)

Currently the subject of much research and popular demand, saw palmetto is a small palm tree native to the southeast coast of North America. An extract of the tree's berries has a long history of medicinal use among Native Americans, who most frequently used it to treat genitourinary problems and to tonify and strengthen the male

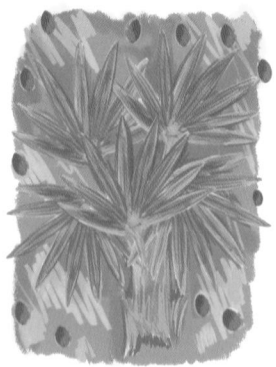

SAW PALMETTO
(Serenoa repens, S. serrulata)

reproductive organs. The berries were also used as an aphrodisiac.

Recent research strongly suggests that saw palmetto is a specific healing agent for BPH, which appears to be caused by an accumulation of testosterone that is in turn converted into a substance called dihydrotestosterone (DHT). DHT seems to overstimulate prostatic cell production, resulting in an enlarged prostate. Saw palmetto's effectiveness against BPH lies in its ability both to inhibit the conversion of testosterone to DHT and to promote the rapid excretion of any DHT, thereby reducing its time in the genitourinary tract. Saw palmetto also has antiseptic and anti-inflammatory actions, making it effective against infections and inflammations. It is also a relaxant, a diuretic, and an expectorant.

Saw palmetto is taken internally for the symptoms of BPH, genitourinary infections, and as a supporting tonic for the male reproductive system. It is available as dried berry pulp and in a variety of commercial preparations, including capsules and teas.

Caution: Minor side effects from overconsumption of saw palmetto may include stomach upset, headaches, and diarrhea. Although saw palmetto was traditionally used to treat female infertility and increase breast size, we do not recommend it for these uses.

Other
Helpful Advice

GO FOR THE GOLD . . . AND GREEN AND RED AND YELLOW!

But avoid the "white"—white rice, white bread, and white pasta from refined grains and flour. A long-term study of over 60,000 American woman found that those who regularly ate refined grains and processed flour had over twice the risk of getting adult-onset (Type II) diabetes than women who ate whole-grain products. They were also at higher risk for heart disease and cancer. Whole grains, on the other hand, which are rich in fiber, essential fatty acids, and free radical-fighting vitamins and minerals such as the B vitamins, vitamin E, calcium, iron, and zinc, are associated with a decreased risk of cancer and heart disease. So too are the immune-boosting, cancer-fighting, carotenoid-loaded green, orange, red, and yellow fruits and vegetables—apples, apricots, carrots, peppers, peaches, spinach, tomatoes, corn, and squash, among others. For optimal health, have 4 or 5 servings of these super-nutritious foods—along with your whole grains—every day.

Strengthening Your Immune System

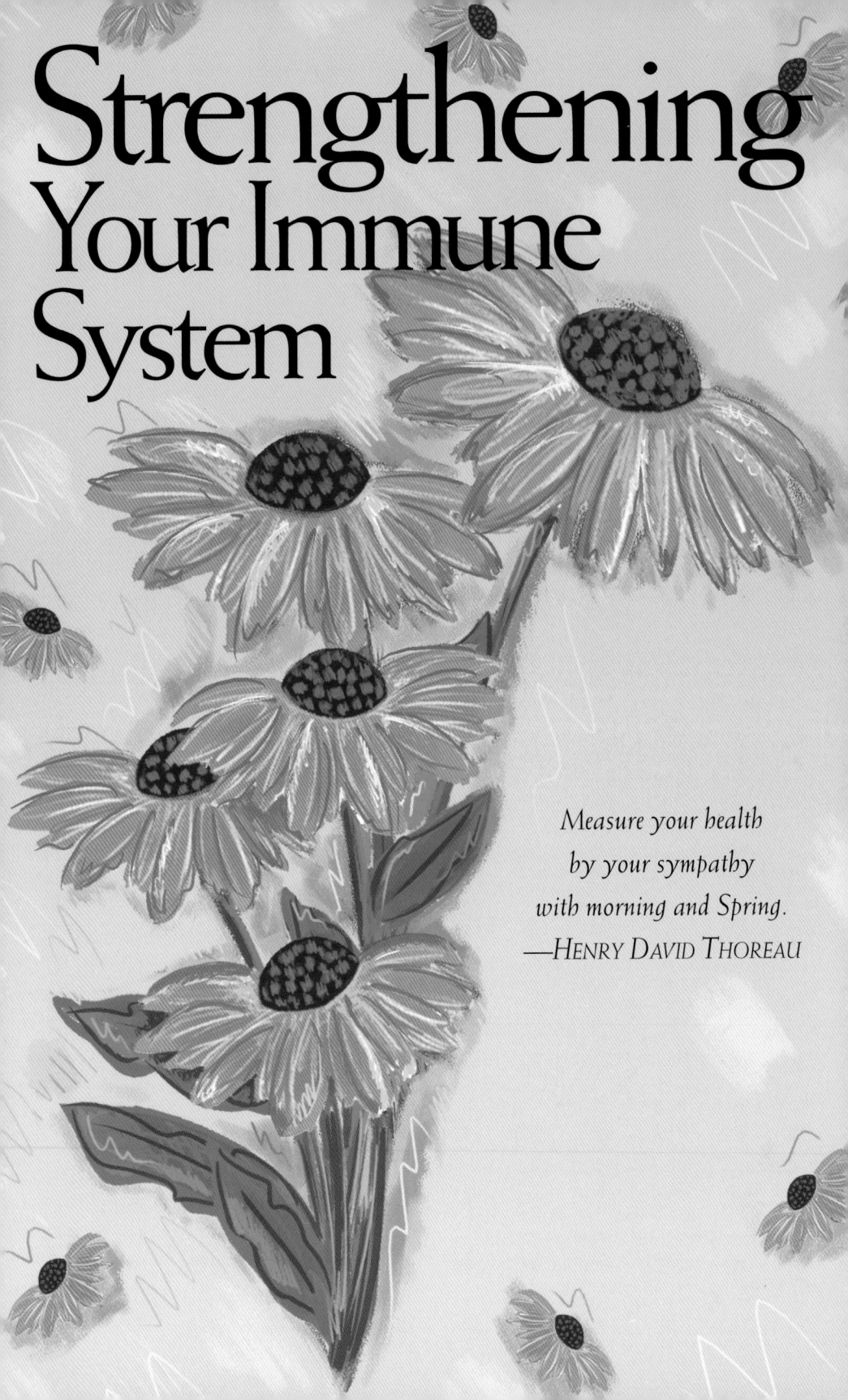

*Measure your health
by your sympathy
with morning and Spring.*
—HENRY DAVID THOREAU

BOOSTING IMMUNITY AND FIGHTING CANCER

Our immune system is an immensely complex entity, the ultimate frontline combat soldier fighting illness, disease, and premature death. Its nonstop job is to search for, identify, and destroy infectious organisms, such as viruses and bacteria. It must also support the body's other systems in inhibiting or destroying cell-damaging toxins, including environmental pollutants and oxidants and free radicals (reactive molecules that can hook up with and damage healthy cells, causing cancerous tumors).

The immune system sometimes fails us in any one of four ways. A temporarily depressed or weakened immune system—often battered by stress or illness—may make the body more susceptible to colds, flu, and other infections. An overactive immune system may turn on the body and attack healthy tissues, mistaking them—for some as toxic agents. This is the cause of many autoimmune diseases, such as rheumatoid arthritis, lupus, and psoriasis. A healthy immune system may overreact to a normally harmless "invader," such as dust, and precipitate an allergic reaction. Lastly, a defect in the immune system that causes it to consistently respond inadequately to toxic and infectious agents is the cause of immunodeficiency diseases such as AIDS.

Many herbs can help support and even stimulate the immune system to function more effectively. Herbs do this by acting as general tonics—nourishing, strengthening, and supporting the body overall. Some herbs function to support the immune system secondarily by treating and regulating major organs, like the liver and kidneys, that are critical to eliminating toxins. Herbs may also directly target the immune system by stimulating the production and metabolism of white blood cells, interferon, macrophages, and phagocytes—all substances that fight viral and bacterial invasion.

Here are some of the best herbs for stimulating and supporting the immune system and for helping prevent the cellular damage that may lead to cancer. Additionally, the herbs listed for treating arthritis and rheumatism (in Chapter 1) and allergies (in Chapter 2) may also be effective for treating immune system problems.

ASTRAGALUS
(Astragalus membranaceus)

Also known as milk vetch root, astragalus root has been used medicinally for thousands of years, first by Chinese herbalists who prized the herb as a superb tonic that nourishes the blood and spleen and is especially effective in treating the lungs. It has also been prescribed by Asian practitioners to help the body fight all manner of illnesses, including viruses and cancers, and to treat diabetes and high blood pressure.

Over the last 15 to 20 years, Western practitioners have similarly prescribed astragalus. Additionally, the herb has been the subject of considerable interest—and ongoing research—for its immune-stimulating and anticancer properties. A number of studies strongly suggest that it has great healing potential in both these areas.

As an immune stimulant, astragalus appears to have several actions. It increases the number of immune cells in the body, thus increasing overall immune system activity; it stimulates dormant immune cells to begin fighting infection; it speeds up the infection-fighting activity of macrophages (cells that attack and consume viruses and bacteria); and it stimulates the production of interferon, a unique cellular protein that also fights infecting organisms.

Astragalus also has a demonstrated immune-stimulating action in people with cancer. It appears to lessen the side effects of chemotherapy, steroid therapy, and radiation, and has been prescribed as a general tonic for patients undergoing chemotherapy. Finally, in several studies, astragalus significantly inhibited the growth of tumors in laboratory mice.

Astragalus is taken internally to stimulate the immune system; for general weakness, fatigue, and loss of appetite; to promote tissue regeneration; to treat blood abnormalities; to prevent chronic colds and flu; and to fight AIDS and cancer (in conjunction with

conventional medical treatments). It is available as dried root, powder, prepared tea, tincture, and capsules.

BARBERRY
(Berberis vulgaris)

We include barberry in this chapter because it is one of the best—yet mildest—of the liver tonics. Also known as sowberry and holy thorn, this relative of Oregon grape has a long history of use by Western herbalists, who have successfully prescribed the root bark to detoxify, nourish, and normalize the liver and liver function. Because the liver is one of the primary organs for cleansing the blood and tissues and helping break down and eliminate toxins from the body, optimal liver function is critical to healthy immune function.

Barberry is also an alterative, one of the family of herbs that acts to strengthen, support, and nourish the body overall, particularly where there is general weakness and debilitation from illness. The herb also contains a potent antibacterial, berberine, which is specifically indicated for a wide range of bacterial infections, including salmonella and streptococcus. It has also been

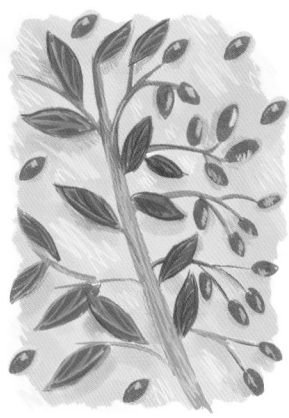

BARBERRY
(Berberis vulgaris)

prescribed for dysentery, diarrhea, gallstones, rheumatism, and conjunctivitis. Many herbalists believe that barberry is also an immune stimulant and anticancer agent.

Taken internally, barberry is available as dried herb, tea, tincture, and capsules. It may also be found in some over-the-counter eyewashes and antidiarrheals.

Caution: Never self-treat a suspected liver problem. Take barberry only on the advice of your medical practitioner and start with the smallest advised dose. An overdose can cause vomiting and a dangerous drop in blood pressure. Barberry is also a uterine tonic, so do not take it if you suspect you are pregnant or you are trying to conceive.

> *Success is never found.*
> *Failure is never fatal.*
> *Courage is the only thing.*
> —Sir Winston Churchill

Blessed Thistle
(Cnicus benedictus)

During the Middle Ages, blessed thistle was regarded as a panacea for a number of ailments and was widely used for treating the plague. Also known as sacred or holy thistle (because of its believed curative powers) and as St. Benedict's thistle (because it was first cultivated at medieval monasteries), blessed thistle was regularly prescribed for centuries as a general tonic, an appetite stimulant, and a treatment for kidney, lung, and liver problems.

Today it is still prescribed as a general tonic and has been variously used to nourish the blood, enhance memory, treat liver dysfunction, heart problems, and cancer, and regulate hormonal imbalances. Viewed by many practitioners as an immune stimu-

lant, blessed thistle, like barberry, is a proven antibacterial. The essential oil found in the flowers destroys several of the staphylococcus bacteria. Blessed thistle's tonifying properties together with its infection-fighting action make it a fine supplemental herb for a weak immune system.

Taken internally, blessed thistle is available as dried herb, tincture, and capsules.

Caution: Blessed thistle has also been used as a contraceptive. Do not take it if you are trying to conceive.

Echinacea
(Echinacea purpurea, E. pallida, E. angustifolia)

In Chapter 2 we discussed echinacea's famed cold- and flu-fighting properties. It acts not only as a preventive agent against infection by cold and flu viruses, but also treats the symptoms of cold and flu when they occur. Taken at the first sign of those symptoms, this native North American plant may even dramatically shorten the course of infection. It is a fine general tonic that nourishes and detoxifies the blood. Echinacea is also a strong anti-inflammatory agent that has been used externally to treat wounds and skin infections and internally to treat arthritis.

Some may view echinacea as a modern wonder drug—along with garlic (for the heart) and St. John's wort (for depression)—but Native Americans used it for centuries for wounds and infections, and its use then spread among European settlers. It became such a popular herbal treatment that it was being used in Europe by the late 1700s.

Also known as the purple coneflower, echinacea's excellent antiviral properties prompted considerable interest from medical researchers, and it has been the subject of more than 350 clinical studies. Many of those studies demonstrate that echinacea is an effective immunostimulant with multiple immune-stimulating actions. The most notable of those is echinacea's ability to stimulate phagocytosis, a critical function of the immune system in which specific cells, such as white blood cells, engulf and destroy invading viruses, bacteria, and other foreign and toxic substances. Like astragalus (discussed earlier in this chapter), echinacea also increases the number of immune cells in the body and stimulates the production of interferon, an important cellular protein that attacks invading organisms.

Several studies also suggest that echinacea may stimulate the production of a protein known as tumor necrosis factor, which inhibits the growth of tumors and thus is critical in the fight against cancer. It also inhibits the production of the bacterial enzyme hyalurinodase, which rapidly spreads infecting bacteria throughout the body.

Taken internally to prevent and treat colds and flu and for its antibiotic and antiviral action, echinacea is also used in the treatment of AIDS and cancer in conjunction with conventional medical treatment. It is now widely available commercially as dried herb, tincture, tea, and capsules (alone or in combination with other herbs).

Caution: If you have HIV, ARC (AIDS-Related Complex), AIDS, or cancer, do not self-treat with echinacea except under the advice of your conventional and alternative practitioners. If you have an autoimmune disease, do not take echinacea without first consulting with a qualified medical practitioner. In some cases of an overactive immune system, an immune stimulant may not be the appropriate choice for treatment.

Recent research suggests that as an immunostimulant, echinacea loses its therapeutic potency with constant daily use. Instead many practitioners suggest that users follow a three-day-on, three-day-off treatment regimen. Other herbalists suggest a week on and a week off. Consult your practitioner about how to take echinacea.

GARLIC
(Allium sativum)

Garlic has proved itself to be a powerful weapon in the fight against heart disease, stroke, and diabetes (see Chapter 4, "Building a Healthy Heart"). It is also a broad-based antibiotic with significant infection-fighting properties against typhoid (for which it is more effective than penicillin), cholera, dysentery, and both the streptococcus and staphylococcus bacteria.

Most recently, researchers have been investigating garlic's anticancer properties. Several studies suggest that garlic appears to inhibit the growth of cancer cells, and it has in fact been successfully used to treat stomach cancer. It may also help prevent the development of breast, throat, and colon cancer.

Garlic is also a potent antioxidant with the ability to neutralize the cell-damaging effects of many environmental pollutants and toxins.

Taken internally for these actions, garlic is available as cloves and in capsules.

Caution: If you have a blood-clotting disorder, consult a qualified practitioner before using garlic.

One must have the adventurous daring to accept oneself as a bundle of possibilities and undertake the most interesting game in the world —making the most of one's best.
—HARRY EMERSON FOSDICK

ASIAN GINSENG
(Panax ginseng)

Growing on the mountains of northeast China, Asian ginseng—or Panax ginseng, as it is more popularly known—is viewed as the most potent of the ginsengs and the greatest of all the "tonic" herbs. In Asian herbal medicine, the root is used to treat an extraordinary number of varied illnesses and ailments, hence its name, Panax, from the Latin *panacea*, which means "cure-all."

Considerable clinical research confirms that Panax ginseng significantly reduces mental and physical fatigue, increases mental clarity, strengthens the body's overall functioning, and helps alleviate the damage caused by physical and emotional stress. These healing properties alone make Asian ginseng a fine herbal supplement for a compromised immune system. (We talk more about Panax ginseng's energy-boosting effects in Chapter 9, "Boosting Your Energy Level.")

Panax ginseng is also what is known as an adaptogen, an herb specifically indicated where there is weakness and debilitation. It appears to be particularly effective in pro-

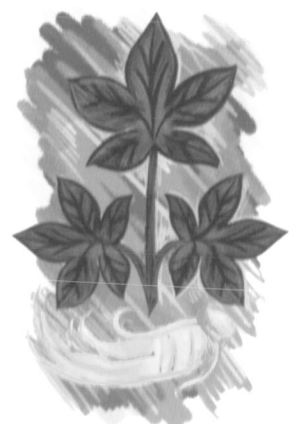

G I N S E N G
(Panax ginseng)

tecting the body against the cellular damage caused by free radicals (invading toxins and pollutants). In that capacity, Panax ginseng greatly supports the functioning of the immune system. It may also regulate and normalize blood sugar and hormone levels and increase the body's ability to deal with stress.

Panax ginseng is taken internally for a damaged immune system, fatigue, stress, viral infections, and inflammatory ailments. It is available as fresh or dried root, powder, capsules, tablets, and tea.

Caution: Always take ginseng under the care of a medical practitioner. Side effects are usually minimal and may include headaches, insomnia, breast soreness, or skin rashes. In some susceptible individuals, however, Panax ginseng may precipitate asthma attacks, increased blood pressure, heart palpitations, or uterine bleeding. If these symptoms occur while you are taking it, consult your practitioner immediately.

SIBERIAN GINSENG
(Eleutherococcus senticosus)

Found in the Siberian region of Russia and in Northern China, Siberian ginseng—or eleuthero, as it is sometimes called—is not, in fact, a true ginseng, though it has long been prized in Asian herbal medicine for its ginseng-like effects. However, like Panax ginseng, Siberian ginseng is a superb tonic and adaptogenic herb, acting to strengthen and normalize all the functions of the body and fight illness, stress, and fatigue. It has a less dramatic effect in these areas than does Asian ginseng, but it is more gentle than the latter and is often used as a substitute because it does not cause the insomnia and jitteriness that Asian ginseng can.

Its primary chemical ingredient, eleutheroside, has been linked repeatedly in research studies to increased stamina, endurance, and athletic performance, garnering Siberian ginseng much popular attention (and use by athletes) and some scientific skepticism, despite supporting clinical evidence by Russian and Japanese researchers. (We discuss Siberian ginseng's effects on memory and mental acuity in Chapter 11, "Sharpening Your Memory.")

There is no doubt about Siberian ginseng's ability to stimulate and support the immune system. It increases both the number and the activity of the white blood cells (lymphocytes) critical to fighting viral infections, and it has repeatedly proved effective in helping prevent stress-induced physical and emotional damage.

Taken internally, Siberian ginseng is available as fresh or dried root, powder, capsules, tablets, and tea. It is often found in combination formulas with ginkgo biloba.

Caution: Talk with your practitioner before taking Siberian ginseng, especially if you have a preexisting medical condition. No appreciable side effects have been reported with its use, although a small number of individuals have experienced insomnia and diarrhea.

Some of your hurts you have cured,
And the sharpest you still
have survived,
But what torments of grief
you endured
From the evil which never arrived.
—RALPH WALDO EMERSON

GRAPE SEED EXTRACT
(*Vitis vinifera*)

We are all familiar with the common grape, long a popular fruit eaten fresh or as raisins and drunk in a variety of wines. Many of us,

however, have never heard about the potent immune-supporting and cancer-fighting potential of the flavonoids extracted from grape seeds.

The most researched and studied of these flavonoids are the oligomeric proanthocyanidins (OPCs), which have proven to be more powerful antioxidants than either vitamins C or E. As an antioxidant, the OPCs help prevent the damage caused by oxidants, free radicals, and invading toxins. They also act as friendly scavengers in the body, engulfing and helping to destroy the same oxidants and free radicals. Both actions support the immune system's work and have potential for helping to prevent cancer.

The antioxidant actions of the OPCs also may help slow down the effects of aging, improve night vision, and treat several eye disorders and vascular ailments, including varicose veins.

Grape seed is available in standardized extracts, most commonly in capsule form. Follow your practitioner's or the manufacturer's directions. No side effects are associated with the consumption of grape seed extract.

GREEN TEA
(*Camellia sinensis*)

Green tea has only recently become popular in the West, but it has been the staple beverage (second only to water) for thousands of years in China and Japan—where the incidence of many cancers is significantly lower than in the West. The tea plant has long been prized in the East as a general tonic with beneficial effects for the entire body.

In fact, green tea is a rich source of the same family (polyphenols) of flavonoid antioxidants found in grape seed extract. This antioxidant action is critical to reducing the effects of damaging free radicals and oxi-

The Perfect Cup of
GREEN TEA

There are many wonderful varieties of green tea commercially available as tea bags. However, if you want to make your own medicinal green tea, use 1 ounce of dried tea or 3 ounces of fresh herb to 1 pint of spring water for each cup of tea made. Bring the water to a boil and then turn off the stove. Place the herbs in a tea pot with lid. Pour the water over the herbs, cover the pot with lid, and allow tea to steep at room temperature for 20 minutes. Strain tea through a small strainer directly into cup. Drink at least 3 cups a day.

dants, which are implicated in the development of many cancers and in accelerated age damage.

Clinical studies have suggested that green tea also reduces total blood cholesterol levels, lowers blood pressure, and acts as an anticlotting agent. Green tea also appears to be a good antibacterial, especially effective against tooth decay and gum disease.

Taken internally as a general tonic, antioxidant, antibacterial, and to treat heart disease, green tea is available as dried leaves and commercially prepared teas. Look for green tea that has been standardized to contain at least 50 percent (and preferably more) polyphenols and at least 50 percent catechins (a special type of polyphenol).

Each day is a little life, every
waking and rising a
little birth, every fresh morning a
little youth, every
going to rest and sleep a little death.
—ARTHUR SCHOPENHAUER

More
Helpful Advice

GET A GOOD NIGHT'S SLEEP—FOR YOUR LIVER'S SAKE.

Traditional Chinese medicine practitioners believe that the liver performs its most vital functions between the hours of 11:00 P.M. and 3:00 A.M. Use the extra energy available while the body sleeps, the liver is especially active replenishing, nourishing, and detoxifying the blood. So if you really want to avoid "tired blood," get to bed by eleven!

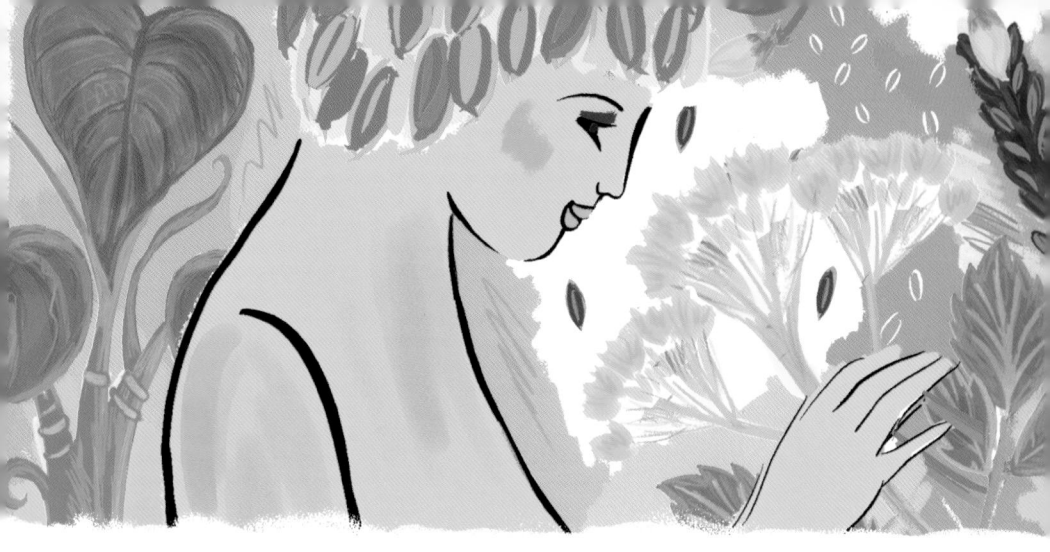

herbs
for
HAPPINESS

"The happiness of life," said the poet Samuel Taylor Coleridge, is found in "the little, soon-forgotten charities of a kiss or smile, a kind look, a heart-felt compliment." Amen. Coleridge's definition of happiness, however old-fashioned, probably rings true for most people. Happiness is rarely found in the obvious claptrap of life, but rather in the quiet places and simple graces shared by people who live and love and work together without any fanfare.

Of course, there are different strokes of happiness for different folks. Dorothy Parker, the wonderfully wicked-tongued, American grande

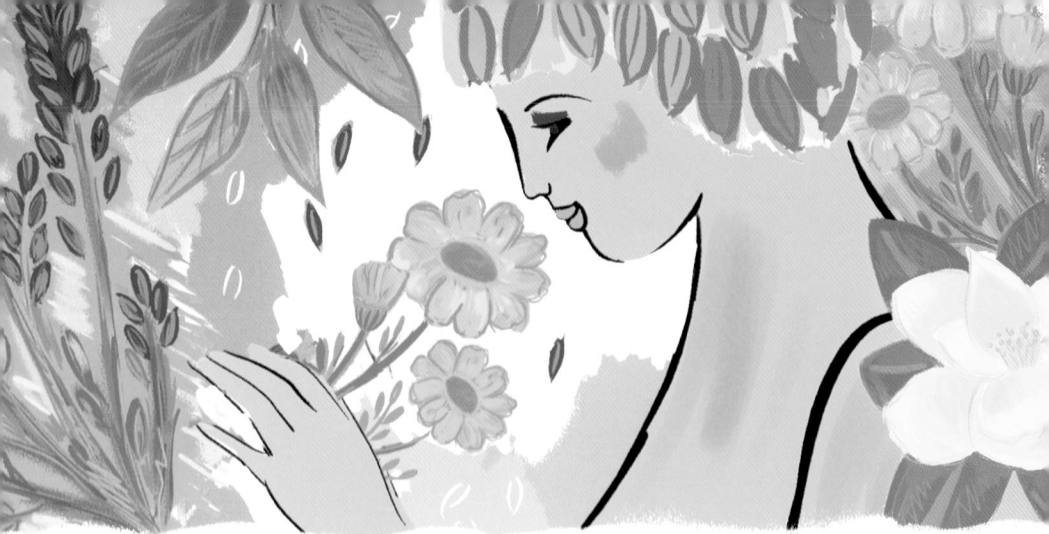

dame of wisecracks, took a much less prosaic tack than Coleridge when it came to personal happiness. Parker once lamented: "Why is it no one ever sent me yet / One perfect limousine, do you suppose? / Ah no, it's always just my luck to get / One perfect rose." And some would say "amen" to that as well. There will always be people for whom happiness can only be measured by the shiny booty of material success.

Happiness is ultimately self-made and sometimes hard-won. Most people build their happiness with equal parts serendipity and sweat. The providential gifts of good health, people to love, and simple comforts, go a long way to sustaining happiness. But when we lose our good health or someone we love; when no amount of simple comforts can assuage the onslaught of overwork, stress, and sleepless nights, reclaiming our happiness may involve hard work.

Can herbs help? Yes and no. There is no magic herbal bullet in all the plant kingdom that will bestow instant happiness on the taker— though some might argue that kava, featured in the next chapter, comes close. What some special herbs can do is nourish, support, and help heal the broken, vulnerable bits of body, mind, and spirit that temporarily fall apart, pushing happiness away. On the following pages we feature such herbs. They can ease anxiety, restore energy, promote good sleep, sharpen the mind, fight depression, and help you feel strong and beautiful. And happy again.

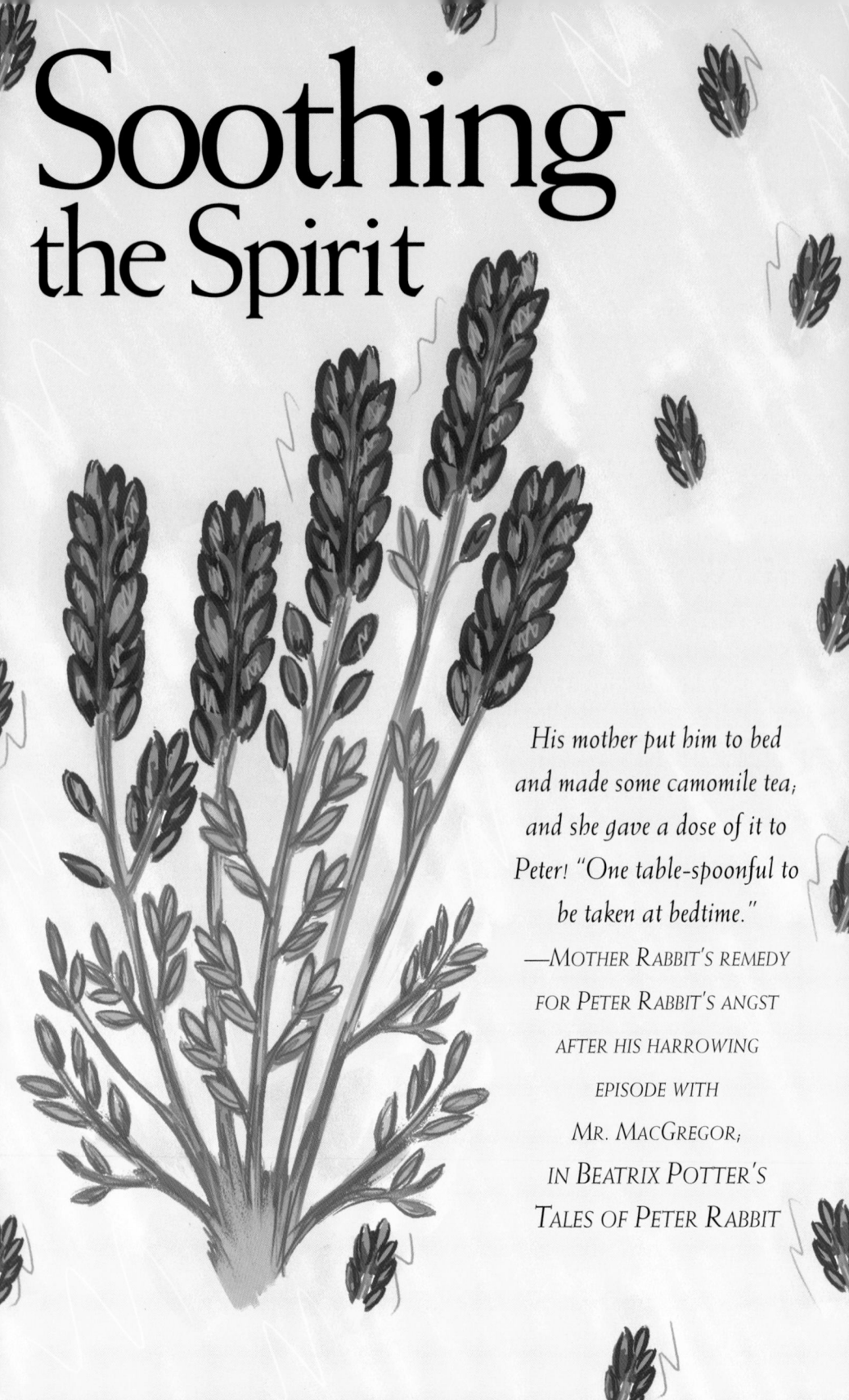

Soothing
the Spirit

*His mother put him to bed
and made some camomile tea;
and she gave a dose of it to
Peter! "One table-spoonful to
be taken at bedtime."*
*—MOTHER RABBIT'S REMEDY
FOR PETER RABBIT'S ANGST
AFTER HIS HARROWING
EPISODE WITH
MR. MACGREGOR,
IN BEATRIX POTTER'S
TALES OF PETER RABBIT*

SLAYING THE SPIRIT DEMONS: ANXIETY, TENSION, AND STRESS

Like three malevolent spirits gathered around the cauldron of our postmodern madness—that roiling brew of too much work, too much stress, too little time, and too little fun—anxiety, tension, and stress collaborate to sap our spirit and sabotage our peace of mind.

Occasional bouts of anxiety or tension or stress are normal of course, and even appropriate: when we change jobs, lose spouses or loved ones, uproot our families, become ill, work too hard and play too little, travel, make speeches, or send children off to college. Chronic anxiety, tension, and stress—that unremitting and near-daily feeling of danger, vulnerability, fear, or unease that never completely leaves us so that we always approach the world in a defensive posture—is not normal and it is downright dangerous to physical and emotional health. The immune system breaks down in the face of chronic stress, making us vulnerable to infection and disease. Unrelieved anxiety and tension not only prevent us from enjoying life; they may lead to incapacitating panic attacks and serious, debilitating depressions.

Were it possible for us to see further than our knowledge reaches, perhaps we would endure our sadnesses with greater confidence than our joys. For they are moments when something new has entered into us, something unknown.
—*RAINER MARIA RILKE*

For the occasional symptoms of anxiety, tension, or stress, many herbs provide effective short-term help. We will present some of the best of those herbs here. Chronic anxiety, tension, and stress, however, need to be treated seriously and carefully with a broad-based approach—usually a combination of professional counseling, lifestyle changes, and medication. The same herbs described here for short-term relief may also be effective (and safer) alternatives to prescription antianxiety and sedating drugs when taken under the care of a qualified practitioner. Additionally, the herbs discussed in Chapter 12, "Fighting the Blues", may also help treat many of the symptoms of anxiety, tension, and stress.

COMMON SYMPTOMS OF ANXIETY, TENSION, AND STRESS

- Fatigue or exhaustion
- Excessive sweating
- Irritability, impatience, and anger
- Rapid or shallow breathing
- Diarrhea or constipation
- Indigestion or nausea
- Insomnia, disturbed sleep, or oversleeping
- Muscle aches and pains and headaches
- Forgetfulness and inability to concentrate
- Chest tightness or discomfort
- Heart palpitations or rapid pulse
- Appetite changes
- Overdrinking

CHAMOMILE
(Matricaria chamomilla [German], Anthemis nobilis [Roman])

Once venerated by the ancient Egyptians because its yellow-and-white daisy-like flowers resembled the sun, chamomile has been used medicinally worldwide for thousands of years. Its common name is derived from the Greek *chamai* ("on the ground") and *melon* ("apple") to mean "ground apple," a dual reference to how the plant grows close to the ground and has a delightful apple scent. In Spain the herb is known as *manzanilla*, or "little apple."

Of the two most common types of chamomile, the most popular and thoroughly studied is German chamomile. Both the Roman and German varieties, however, have similar therapeutic properties, although the German chamomile makes a better tea. (The Roman plant is somewhat bitter tasting.) Both conventional researchers and modern herbalists have identified elements in the oil of the chamomile flower—primarily apigenin and azulene—

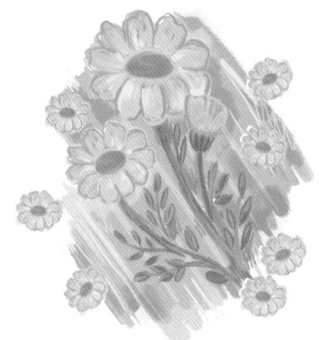

CHAMOMILE
(Matricaria chamomilla [German], Anthemis nobilis [Roman])

that appear to calm the central nervous system, relax the digestive tract, speed healing, and fight infectious bacteria. Chamomile is also rich in calcium, magnesium, and iron. The warm tea is wonderfully calming and helps induce relaxation and promote sleep. Soaking in a chamomile bath will not only calm frazzled nerves; it may relieve minor aches and pains.

Taken internally—famously so in teas—chamomile also has sedating, antispasmodic, pain-relieving, and wound-healing properties. It is additionally prescribed for ulcers, gas, nervous stomach, indigestion, and menstrual cramps. Some holistic practitioners have even used it to treat attention deficit disorder. Chamomile is available as dried or fresh flowers, prepared tea, tincture, and essential oil. It is often found in commercially prepared teas mixed with other herbs and used for both relaxation and sleep. It combines especially well with kava kava, valerian, and passionflower.

Caution: Allergies to chamomile are rare, but individuals allergic to other plants in the daisy, ragweed, aster, and chrysanthemum families should be alert to possible allergic reactions to chamomile.

KAVA KAVA
(Piper methysticum)

This "latest" and most popular of the stress-busting herbs is native to the Melanesia and Polynesia islands in the South Pacific. There the root of the plant is made into an intoxicating, relaxing tea used in many island ceremonies. Kava, as it is also known, only seems like the latest herb to attract popular and scientific attention. In fact, this member of the pepper family has been used in the West for more than 200 years, ever

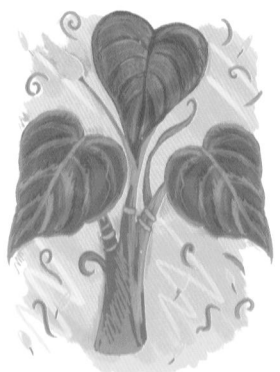

KAVA KAVA
(Piper methysticum)

since James Cook, the celebrated eighteenth-century British explorer, brought the plant back to Europe.

Researchers first began looking into the relaxant properties of kava in the 1950s, but only recently have clinical studies strongly suggested that kava is truly unique among the herbs that treat anxiety and stress. Most antianxiety agents—especially conventional drugs, such as Valium and other benzodiazepines—produce a calming effect by blocking (binding to) specific brain chemical sites that affect emotions. However, the same binding action that results in feeling calmer can dull other senses, especially mental alertness. Kava, at prescribed doses, is unique because it appears to modify rather than block these same brain chemicals, resulting in an unusual combination of elevated mood; calm, meditative state; and increased mental alertness. Kava is also an excellent muscle relaxant with pain-relieving properties, making it an effective treatment for musculoskeletal tension, pain, and spasm; menstrual cramps; and arthritic pain. It is also prescribed for insomnia and headache.

The plant chemicals responsible for kava's effectiveness are called kavalactones, and they are extracted from the plant's roots. Commercial preparations of kava are standardized to range in potency from 3 percent to 30 percent kavalactones; that is, from the mildest sedating action to the most potent sedating effects. Check with your practitioner about the best dosage and potency for you.

Taken internally, kava is available as dried root, tincture, tea, and capsules. In teas it is often combined with other calming herbs, such as chamomile, lavender, and passionflower.

Caution: Take kava only at recommended doses (follow your practitioner's or the manufacturer's directions) for no longer than three months at a time, unless you are under medical advice. High doses of kava or extended self-treatment may cause skin, hair, and nail discoloration; scaly skin; swollen face and eyes; muscle weakness; and motor and vision problems. Avoid alcohol when taking kava and be cautious about driving or operating machinery until you are used to the herb's effects.

Do not take kava with conventional anti-anxiety drugs or sleep medications to avoid possible oversedation of the central nervous system. Do not take kava if you have been diagnosed with depression or if you have Parkinson's disease.

A day dawns,
quite like other days;
in it, a single hour comes,
quite like other hours;
but in that day and in that hour
the chance of a lifetime faces us.
—MALTBIE BABCOCK

LAVENDER
(*Lavandula officinalis*)

One of the most distinctively aromatic of the healing herbs, lavender has a long and famous history of commercial and medicinal use. Widely used in soaps, bath products, perfumes, powders, sachets, and moth repellents, it is easy to forget that lavender also has proven therapeutic properties. Herbalists prescribe lavender tea (taken internally) and the essential oil of lavender (used externally) to treat common emotional stress, tension, insomnia, headache, and nausea. Many herbalists believe that lavender is a gentle, nourishing tonic for the central nervous system and an effective weapon against emotional damage caused by chronic stress and anxiety.

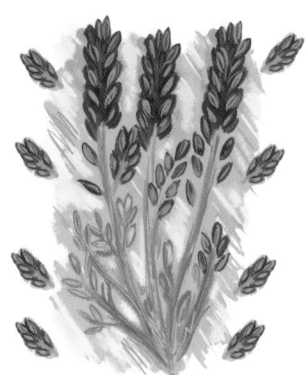

LAVENDER
(*Lavandula officinalis*)

Long a staple in aromatherapy treatment, lavender's essential oil is used to promote relaxation, stimulate the mind, clarify thinking, encourage creativity, and help relieve depression.

Taken internally for emotional stress and tension; depression; insomnia; and stress-related headaches, muscle aches, indigestion, nausea, and flatulence, lavender is available as dried flowers, powdered herb, tea, capsules, tincture, and essential oil. Follow your practitioner's or the manufacturer's directions. In teas, lavender is often combined with rosemary, skullcap, or kola nut to treat the symptoms of depression.

Caution: Never use lavender oil internally.

SKULLCAP/SCUTE
(*Scutellaria baicalensis*)

The skullcap species, commonly known as scute in the West and huang qin in China, has a long history of use among Asian herbalists. They prescribe decoctions of the root for a variety of ailments, including diarrhea, respiratory and urinary tract infections, high blood pressure, headache, nosebleeds, and the symptoms of premenstrual syndrome. It is an especially effective herb for normalizing liver function.

Scute is also frequently prescribed for tension, nervousness, irritability, and insomnia; it may often be combined in herbal formulas with angelica sinensis, gentian, or turmeric. Available in herbal formulas and as dried herb in Asian pharmacies and markets, and in commercial health food stores, scute may also be obtained in capsules.

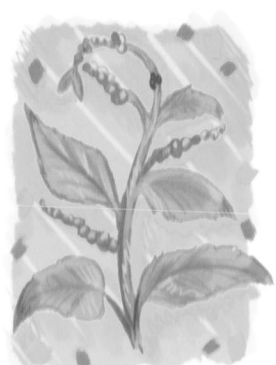

SKULLCAP/SCUTE
(*Scutellaria baicalensis*)

> *Everything has its wonders,*
> *even darkness and silence,*
> *and I learn, whatever state*
> *I may be in, therein to be content.*
> —HELEN KELLER

SKULLCAP/VIRGINIAN
(*Scutellaria lateriflora*)

The leaves and blue flowers of the Virginian species of skullcap have long been used in many herbal sleep remedies and tranquilizing teas. Native Americans regularly used skullcap as a sedative and indigestion treatment. In Eastern traditional herbal medicine, it is often prescribed for hepatitis, as it has the same liver-normalizing properties as scute (see earlier).

In the United States, the use of skullcap—once unpopularly known as mad-dog weed—was long viewed as controversial and even useless, due in part to its early and undeserved reputation as a cure for rabies. In truth, skullcap is a proven sedative, antispasmodic, and nervine. Herbal nervines can calm and sedate; relieve muscle pain, tension, and spasm; and act to nourish and normalize the central nervous system. Some holistic practitioners believe that skullcap is particularly effective in neutralizing negative emotions (like anger and hatred) and helping to enhance the meditative state.

Taken internally, skullcap is also effectively used to ease drug or alcohol withdrawal. It is available as dried herb, tea, tincture, and capsules. The hot tea is especially effective in treating anxiety and tension.

Caution: Use skullcap only under the supervision of a qualified practitioner. Side effects may include stomach upset or diarrhea. Reduce your intake or stop usage if

A Breath of
SERENITY

Aromatherapists believe that inhaling the essential oil of lavender has a stabilizing effect on the whole psyche, helping to dispel emotional stress; promote a calm, relaxed state; and sharpen intuition and creative instincts. After a particularly trying day, when you need to "regroup" emotionally, heat 3 to 6 drops of lavender oil in a diffuser, place in your room, put your feet up, and simply breathe.

these side effects occur. Taking large amounts of skullcap may produce confusion, giddiness, twitching, and convulsions. Skullcap may also cause drowsiness. Be cautious when driving or operating heavy machinery.

No longer forward nor behind
I look in hope or fear;
But, grateful, take the good I find,
The best of now and here.
—*JOHN GREENLEAF WHITTIER*

VALERIAN
(*Valeriana officinalis*)

Used worldwide for more than 1,000 years as a relaxant, valerian root is often thought of as the "Valium" of the plant kingdom. In fact, it is not chemically related at all to that famously overprescribed pharmaceutical. Recent research does confirm, however, that valerian is indeed a mild and safe

tranquilizer that is particularly useful for treating anxiety, nervous tension, stress, and panic attacks. Valerian also helps promote a good night's sleep—by hastening sleep's onset and reducing nighttime awakenings—without interfering with the dreaming or rapid eye movement stage of sleep as do pharmaceutical sedatives and sleep aids. Most people who use valerian also report no morning "hangover" or grogginess, although this effect—or lack thereof—is still under debate. Valerian is considered non-habit-forming and produces no withdrawal symptoms when discontinued. Nevertheless, it must only be taken at prescribed dosages.

Valerian is taken internally for anxiety, nervousness, and tension; stress-related headache, muscle ache, and intestinal pains; menstrual cramps; and insomnia. It is available as dried herb, capsules, tincture, and teas, alone or in combination with many other calming herbs, including St. John's wort, hops, passionflower, and kava kava.

Caution: Take valerian only at minimal prescribed dosages. Minor side effects may include a mild headache or upset, but more serious side effects—almost always related

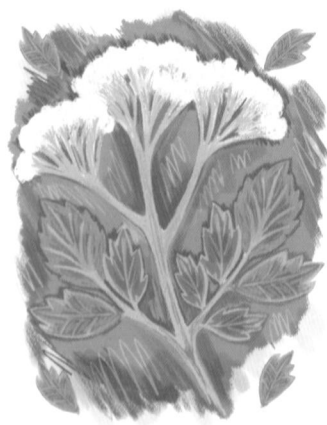

VALERIAN
(Valeriana officinalis)

to overconsumption of the herb—may include severe headache, restlessness, nausea, morning grogginess, or blurred vision. An overdose of valerian may dangerously weaken the heartbeat. Contact your practitioner if you experience any of these side effects.

Do not take valerian with conventional tranquilizers or sedatives because of possible increased effects. Be cautious about driving or operating machinery until you know how the herb affects you.

You are used to listening
to the buzz of the world,
but now is the time to develop
the inner ear that listens
to the inner world.
It is time to have a foot
in each world, and it can be done.
—ST. BARTHOLOMEW

More Helpful Advice

SUPER STRESS-BUSTERS: STRETCHING AND WALKING

To help relieve the symptoms of stress—as well as improve your body's flexibility and strengthen your heart—make room in your life for a daily routine of stretching and walking. Fifteen minutes of gentle neck, back, waist, and leg stretches, followed by 30 minutes of brisk walking will diminish the effects of stress by re-energizing your body, soothing your spirits, and settling your thoughts.

Boosting Your Energy Level

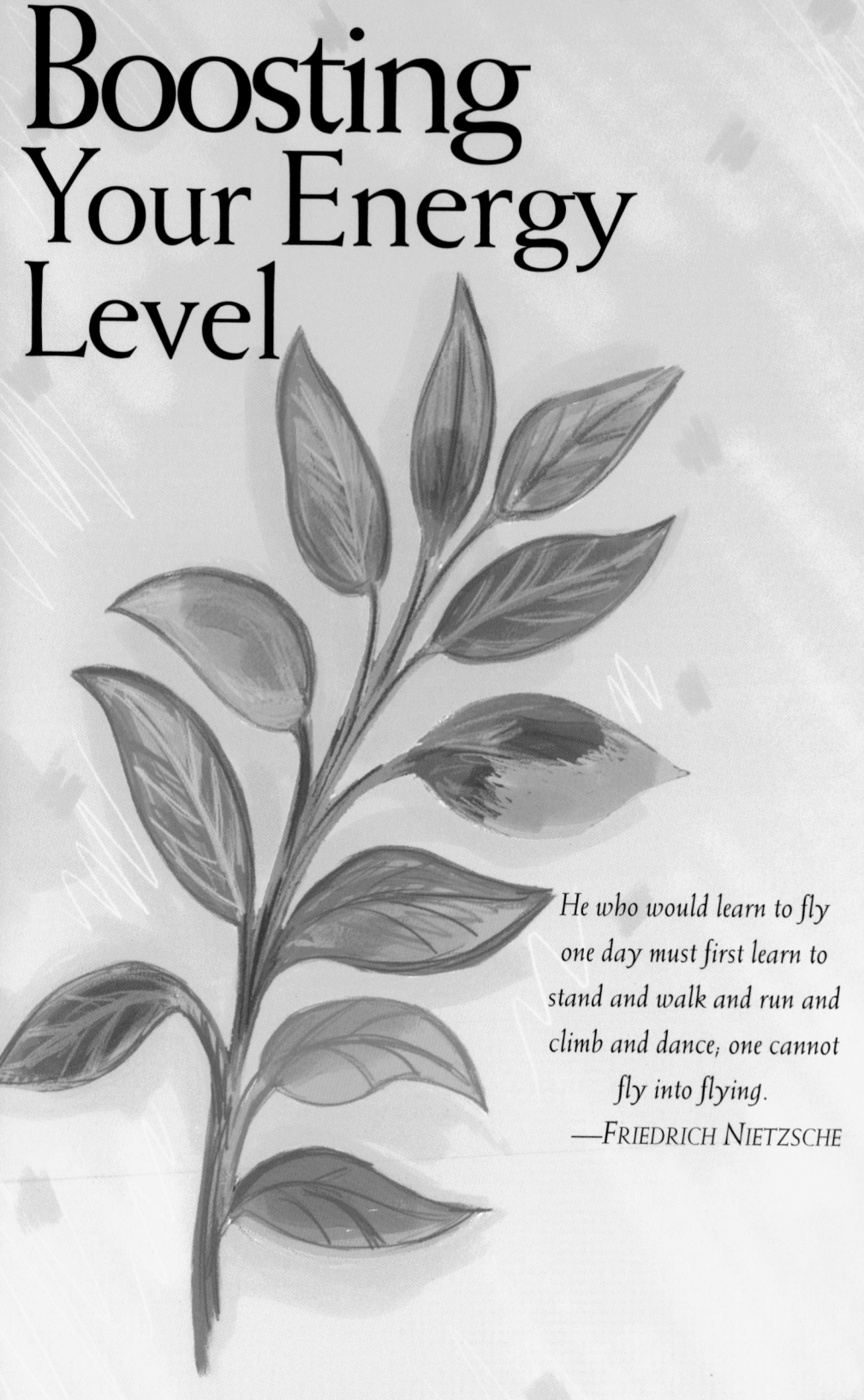

He who would learn to fly one day must first learn to stand and walk and run and climb and dance; one cannot fly into flying.
—FRIEDRICH NIETZSCHE

RESTARTING YOUR ENGINES

Exhaustion, fatigue, and low energy—like their near cousins, anxiety, tension, and stress—are often by-products of our lifestyles. Overwork, poor diets, little exercise, and insufficient sleep will gradually take their toll on body and soul. Exhaustion, chronic fatigue, and little energy are not only physically debilitating and emotionally draining, they are often the first signs that we're not taking good care of ourselves. And while they are serious problems in and of themselves, they may be harbingers of more serious problems to come—if we don't reexamine and readjust our often harried and haphazard lives.

Exhaustion, fatigue, and a lack of energy may also be symptoms of any number of medical conditions—poor or obstructed blood circulation, cancer, diabetes, heart disease, hepatitis, and hypothyroidism (underactive thyroid), to name just a few. If your exhaustion, fatigue, and poor energy have become chronic, it's essential that you have a qualified practitioner check for any underlying illness. Having done that, many herbs offer support for the terminally tired by acting as tonics, restoratives, and stimulants. The following are some of the finest.

It isn't important to come out on top;
what matters is to be
the one who comes out alive.
—BERTOLT BRECHT

ANGELICA SINENSIS/ DONG QUAI
(*Angelica sinensis*)

Chinese herbal medicine's premiere restorative "female" tonic is particularly effective in relieving exhaustion, low energy, and other debilitative symptoms which are caused by hormonal problems and imbalances, including those associated with menstrual problems and menopause. As one of the finest blood-nourishing tonics, angelica sinensis is also very effective in treating anemia, one of the prime causes of fatigue and exhaustion in women and men. (For more information on angelica sinensis, see Chapter 5, "Calming an Upset Stomach.")

Also known as Chinese angelica root and tang gui, angelica sinensis normalizes, nourishes, and supports the overall functioning of the body and promotes healthy blood circulation, two actions which can increase stamina and energy levels. Among its many other clinically-confirmed tonifying actions are the ability to lower blood pressure, slow the pulse rate, relax the heart muscle, and stabilize blood sugar levels. Angelica sinensis additionally has sedating, analgesic, and calming effects.

Taken internally as a blood tonic and for the fatigue and exhaustion associated with menstrual complaints, menopause, anemia, and other blood and hormonal imbalances, angelica sinensis may also be prescribed for heart palpitations and constipation. It is available as dried herb, tea, tincture, and capsules.

Caution: Do not use this herb if you have diarrhea or abdominal bloating. Consult your medical practitioner instead.

> *To burn always with this*
> *hard gemlike flame. To maintain*
> *this ecstasy, is success in life.*
> —*WALTER PATER*

DAMIANA
(Turnera diffusa, T. aphrodisiaca)

The leaves of this aromatic perennial smell much like chamomile, but damiana—also known as Mexican damiana and *Turnera*—is rarely used as a calming herb (though it does have some relaxant effects). Instead, damiana tea, made from the leaves and stems of the plant, is first and foremost a mild stimulant (at prescribed doses), and one with a particular attraction for reproductive organ tissue—the reason for the

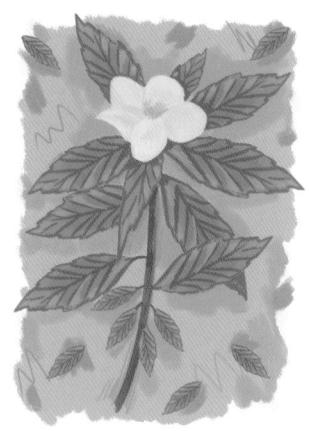

DAMIANA
(Turnera diffusa, T. aphrodisiaca)

herb's longtime reputation as an aphrodisiac. The combination of alkaloids in damiana's chemical makeup are believed to have a testosterone-like effect on genitourinary mucous membranes, and the herb has been used to treat both male and female sexual dysfunction, including impotence and low

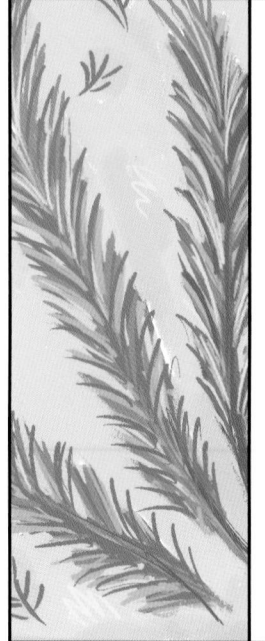

Essential Oils that

ENERGIZE BODY, MIND, AND SOUL

Inhaling the essential oils of rosemary, orange, melissa, and jasmine stimulates and rejuvenates the body, mind, and spirit. Combine 3 drops of each oil in a diffuser and allow their intoxicating aromas to fill a room. For a stimulating and sensual bath, stir the same quantity of combined oils into a warm bath and simmer yourself for at least 20 minutes.

sex drive. (Increased levels of testosterone are linked to increased sex drive.) The same alkaloids also act as mildly euphoric stimulants with effects similar to those of caffeine.

In Mexico, where damiana is a native plant (as it is in Texas and Central America), damiana tea has a long history of medicinal use, most notably as a restorative tonic for the central nervous system—a proven therapeutic use for which it is frequently prescribed today. Damiana appears to be particularly effective in treating the symptoms of general debilitation, including exhaustion and low energy, when emotional stress may be a contributing factor. It may also be used as a laxative and may have antidepressant properties.

Damiana is taken internally to strengthen and tonify the central nervous and hormonal system; to increase stamina; to treat sexual dysfunction; and to relieve the exhaustion and lethargy associated with general debilitation. It may also be prescribed for anxiety, depression, and genital herpes. Anecdotal information suggests that damiana is also an aphrodisiac. It is available as dried herb, tincture, and tea.

Caution: Take damiana only at prescribed doses and only for its therapeutic effects. Damiana should not be used as a "recreational drug." Overconsumption or abuse of the herb may result in serious overstimulation of the central nervous system. Do not take damiana if you have a manic-depressive disorder or irritable bowel syndrome, or if you have been diagnosed as hyperactive.

Vigor is contagious, and whatever makes us either think or feel strongly adds to our power and enlarges our field of action.
—RALPH WALDO EMERSON

GINGER
(Zingiber officinale)

Ginger has so many therapeutic properties that entire books have been written about this tropical herb, and it could easily be featured in just about every chapter in this book. It is variously and successfully prescribed as an antibiotic, antispasmodic, analgesic, and antioxidant, and is useful for treating nausea, vomiting, sore throats, colds, flu, bronchitis, aches and pains, indigestion, flatulence, diarrhea, high cholesterol, and blood-clotting disorders.

Like damiana (described earlier), ginger even has an anecdotal reputation as an aphrodisiac. That reputation is due in part to the fact that ginger, again like damiana, is a potent stimulant. It increases blood circulation, stimulates the body's metabolism, raises energy levels, and combats fatigue and exhaustion.

Ginger is available as fresh or dried root, tincture, capsules, and prepared tea. It is often combined—in teas and capsules—with restorative and tonifying herbs, such as ginkgo and ginseng. It is a very safe herb; only mild side effects, heartburn is one, have been reported.

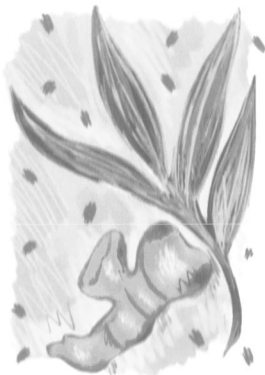

GINGER
(Zingiber officinale)

CAFFEINE:
A LITTLE GOES
A LONG WAY...

Caffeine often gets an undeservedly bad rap, mostly because Americans abuse this natural energizer. We tend to overconsume black coffee (at 90 mg of caffeine per cup!) and that's in addition to those double espressos (at 160 mg of caffeine per cup) that we linger over in sidewalk cafes. Too much caffeine taxes the urinary and digestive systems, dehydrates the body, and, rather than relieving fatigue, causes a "rebound" crash of exhaustion later in the day. But using caffeine responsibly—up to four, 8-ounce cups a day—can provide a natural energizing boost, clear the mind, promote concentration, and even relieve aches and pains. The many robustly flavored and aromatic black teas—Kenyan and Assam are two of the best—contain only 60 mg of caffeine per cup and provide a delicious, and just as energizing, alternative to coffee.

GINSENG
(Panax ginseng [Asian], Eleutherococcus sentiosus [Siberian], Panax quinquefolium [Native American])

All three ginsengs—even the Siberian, which technically isn't a real ginseng—are superlative tonics, restoratives, and stimulants. The ginsengs have many therapeutic benefits, but they are most esteemed for strengthening and nourishing the body, increasing stamina, and restoring energy levels. Having said that, each ginseng does have its own unique strengths, which we highlight here.

ASIAN GINSENG. This most potent—and expensive—of the ginsengs is renowned for its ability to strengthen the immune system and increase the body's ability to deal with fatigue and stress. Herbalists prescribe Asian ginseng to nourish both the body and mind and restore vitality when the body is compromised by chronic illness, debilitation, or old age. It is used to increase blood circulation, support new tissue growth, stimulate the appetite, and help the body fight off infectious viruses and bacteria.

Taken internally for depression, fatigue, stress, and a compromised immune system, Asian ginseng is available as fresh, dried, or freeze-dried root, root powder, capsules, tablets, and prepared tea. Follow your practitioner's directions for dosage and duration of treatment.

Even if you're on the right track, you'll get run over if you just sit there.
—WILL ROGERS

Caution: Use only under the direction of an herbalist or a healthcare professional if you have insomnia, hay fever, fibrocystic breasts, asthma, emphysema, high blood pressure, blood-clotting or heart disorders, or diabetes. Minor side effects may include headache, insomnia, anxiety, breast soreness, or skin rash. Serious side effects include asthma attacks, increased blood pressure, heart palpitations, or postmenopausal uterine bleeding. If any of these symptoms occur, stop using ginseng and consult your doctor.

SIBERIAN GINSENG. Found in the Siberian regions of Russia and in northern China, Siberian ginseng—also called eleuthero—has many of the same medicinal properties as Asian ginseng but the overall therapeutic effect is subtler and less intense. This makes it a particularly good tonic—as a tea or made into a wine—for the chronically ill and the elderly. Conversely, it is also used by athletes, pilots, and nightshift workers, among others, for its famous ability to increase endurance, energy, and stamina. Repeated clinical studies demonstrate that Siberian ginseng significantly improves athletic performance and greatly speeds up recovery time after exertion. Siberian ginseng is also notable for not causing the insomnia and jitteriness that sometimes occur with Asian and Native American ginsengs.

Taken internally for fatigue, stress, depression, and a damaged immune system, and to increase energy, endurance, stamina, and athletic performance, Siberian ginseng is available as fresh, dried, or freeze-dried root, root powder, capsules, tablets, and prepared tea. Follow your practitioner's directions for dosage and duration of treatment.

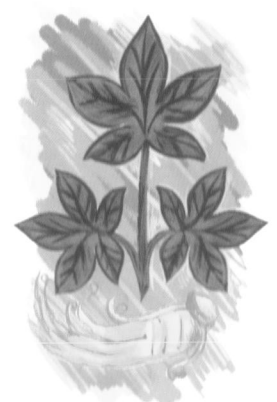

G I N S E N G

(Panax ginseng [Asian],
Eleutherococcus sentiosus [Siberian],
Panax quinquefolium [Native American])

> *As the soft yield of water cleaves*
> *obstinate stone, So to yield with life*
> *solves the insolvable: To yield,*
> *I have learned, is to*
> *come back again.*
> *—LAO-TZU*

Caution: See Asian ginseng for cautions and contraindications.

NATIVE AMERICAN GINSENG. Native Americans used American ginseng to lessen the pain of childbirth and increase energy in the elderly. Two of the most active ingredients in American ginseng are the panaxosides, which are believed to calm the brain and act as a mild stimulant, and germanium, which may be one of the agents responsible for American ginseng's remarkable ability to effectively and gently treat the physical and mental symptoms of chronic weakness, debilitation, and immune dysfunction. It is milder than Asian ginseng and often prescribed for people who consider the latter too potent. Native American ginseng is considered an endangered species because of excessive harvesting.

Taken internally as a tonic for depression, fatigue, stress, and a compromised immune system, Native American ginseng is also particularly effective in treating the fevers, night sweats, coughs (with or without bleeding), and respiratory problems which may accompany many chronic debilitating conditions, including AIDS. Native American ginseng is available as fresh, dried, or freeze-dried root, root powder, capsules, tablets, and prepared tea. Follow your practitioner's directions for dosage and duration of treatment.

Caution: See Asian ginseng for cautions and contraindications.

KELP/BLADDERWRACK
(*Fucus vesiculosus, Fucus species*)

One of the many species of seaweed, kelp was the original source of iodine, first discovered in the early 1800s and used for the next 50 years to treat goiter (enlargement of the thyroid gland, which regulates the body's metabolism).

Also popularly known as bladderwrack (for its familiar, bladder-like "bubbles") and rockweed (because it clings to tidal rocks and stones), the *Fucus* species of kelp and the *Laminaria* species (a much larger seaweed, also called kelp) are not only great sources of iodine, they are rich in potassium, calcium, magnesium, vitamins A and C, and the B-vitamin complex. Additionally, they contain large amounts of essential trace minerals such as selenium, manganese, and phosphorus.

> *What you can do, or dream you can do, begin it; boldness has genius, power and magic in it.*
> —JOHANN WOLFGANG VON GOETHE

If that isn't inducement enough to add seaweed to your diet, kelp is also a well-known and very effective stimulant and weight-loss aid. Those are secondary effects of kelp's main therapeutic actions: regulating the thyroid gland which in turn stimulates the body's metabolism, raises energy levels, and relieves fatigue. Herbalists prescribe kelp to treat hypothyroidism (an underactive and sluggish thyroid) and the obesity which accompanies it. Not surprisingly, kelp is frequently part of many weight-loss programs. It is also an important preventative against the effects of

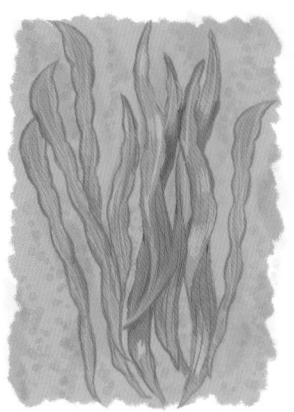

KELP/BLADDERWRACK
(*Fucus vesiculosus*)

environmental and heavy-metal pollutants on the body.

Taken internally for goiter, hypothyroidism, and obesity, kelp is available in dry bulk, powered herb, capsules, and tincture.

Caution: If you are already taking medication for hyperthyroidism (overactive thyroid), kelp supplements could worsen the condition. Do not gather your own fresh kelp; coastal colonies may be contaminated by offshore pollutants. Check with your local environmental agency about safe harvesting locales. Kelp is very high in sodium, so consult with your practitioner before using kelp if you have a history of high blood pressure; also check with your practitioner if you have or have had thyroid problems or thyroid cancer.

SAGE
(*Salvia officinalis*)

A centuries-old herb which was once believed to be a lifesaving panacea for all that ails humankind (the Latin *salvia* means "healing plant" and is derived from *salvere*, which means "to save"), sage's many medicinal uses are legion indeed. While it is known today more as a culinary herb, over the centuries herbalists have prescribed sage for asthma, diarrhea, eczema, gingivitis, cholera, colds, constipation, indigestion, infertility, sore throats, ulcers, and wounds! As one ancient proverb says, "How can a man die who has sage in his garden?"

Common sage, as *Salvia officinalis* is popularly called, contains the most medicinal properties. There are many other varieties of sage, however, some of which are strictly culinary or decorative, and others of which have quite specific medicinal uses: Clary sage (*Salvia sclarea*) is used as a digestive aid, an eyewash, and as a stimulating bath; painted sage (*Salvia horminum*) is used as a gargle for sore throats.

Two of common sage's most famous therapeutic benefits—ones for which it is still prescribed today—are as a central nervous system tonic and a circulatory stimulant. It is specifically prescribed to treat the fatigue, exhaustion, and general debilitation associated with recovery from serious illness and with depression and severe stress. Three cups a day of sage tea is traditionally prescribed to maintain optimal health.

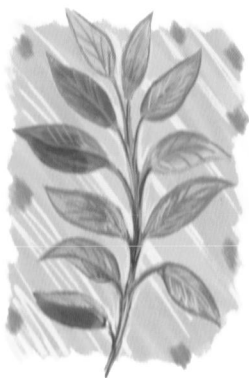

S A G E
(*Salvia officinalis*)

Taken internally as a tonic and stimulant, sage is available as fresh or dried herb, tincture, tea, and oil.

Caution: Fresh sage contains the toxic chemical thujone, which can lead to convulsions if taken in high doses. If you use fresh sage to make a tea, always steep the herb in boiling water; heat reduces thujone's toxicity. Never ingest sage oil, and do not take the herb in any form if you have epilepsy or you are nursing.

HAVING YOUR SEAWEED and Eating It Too

If the thought of eating seaweed makes you gag, you are among the majority of Americans. But you are in a decided minority when it comes to the rest of the world. In countries as diverse as Ireland, Japan, Denmark, Iceland, China, and Wales, seaweed is a staple food product, eaten fresh and in salads, soups, and vegetable dishes. If you're interested in learning how to cook with seaweed, Judith Madlener's *The Sea Vegetable Book* (Clarkson N. Potter Publishing, 1977) contains over 200 seaweed recipes.

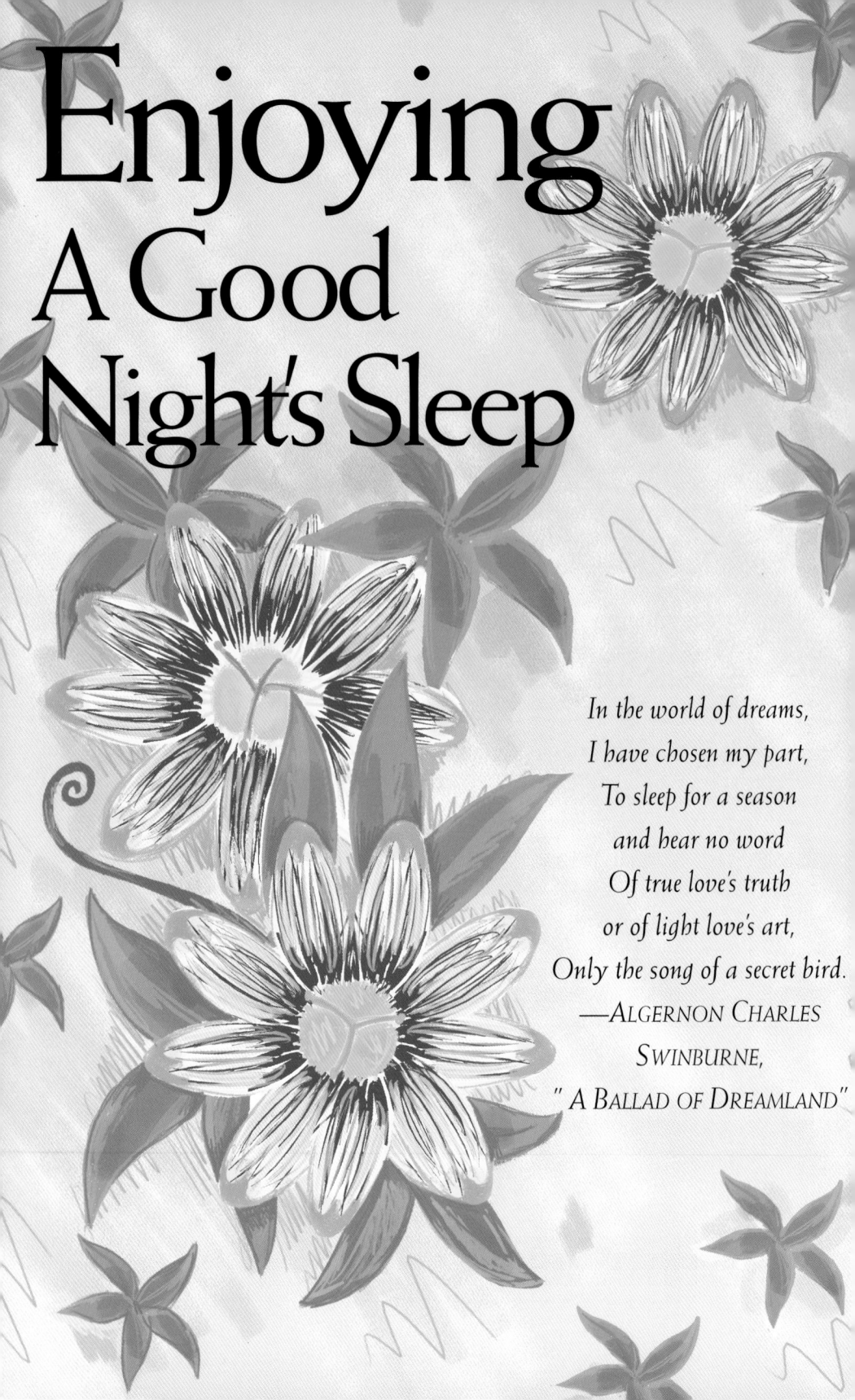

Enjoying
A Good
Night's Sleep

In the world of dreams,
I have chosen my part,
To sleep for a season
and hear no word
Of true love's truth
or of light love's art,
Only the song of a secret bird.
—ALGERNON CHARLES
SWINBURNE,
" A BALLAD OF DREAMLAND"

TO SLEEP . . .

More than 30 percent of Americans suffer from insomnia and other sleep disorders. Overwork, irregular work hours, fast food, lack of exercise, too much stress and worry, and too little time to relax are just some of the reasons people experience intermittent bouts of insomnia. Sleep disturbances, including insomnia, can also be the result of underlying physical, mental, or emotional conditions or a side effect of some medications.

Insomnia is usually defined as inadequate or disturbed sleep, and it includes one or more of the following symptoms: difficulty falling asleep, inability to sleep through the night, repeatedly waking up throughout the night, restless and insufficient sleep, waking up too early, and waking up feeling exhausted. Insomnia and disturbed sleep are further defined as either transient (lasting just a few nights), short-term (lasting just a few weeks), or chronic (persisting for more than three weeks).

The effects of transient and short-term sleep disorders—however intermittent and short-lived—can still seriously affect work performance, emotional health, and family and personal relationships. Some of those effects include daytime drowsiness, anxiousness, irritability, inability to concentrate, and decreased motor skills. These effects are greatly intensified with chronic insomnia, which, untreated, can wreak havoc with one's personal and professional lives and jeopardize physical health and emotional well-being. Chronic insomnia should always be evaluated and treated by a qualified practitioner.

Many herbs hold a time-honored place in the treatment of transient and short-term sleep disorders. Sedating herbs can help promote good sleep by relaxing and calming the body and mind. Other herbs appear to act directly as hypnotics or soporifics, inducing a deep, restful sleep without interfering with normal dream patterns or causing the morning sluggishness and headache that are frequent side effects of pharmaceutical sleep aids.

All of the herbs highlighted in Chapter 8 "Soothing the Spirit" for their calming effects on body and spirit are also helpful in promoting a good night's sleep. In fact, they are often combined in teas and herbal formulas with the excellent sleep-inducing herbs featured here.

Stars of the summer night!
Far in yon azure deeps
Hide, hide your golden light!
She sleeps! my lady sleeps!
—HENRY WADSWORTH LONGFELLOW
"THE SPANISH STUDENT"

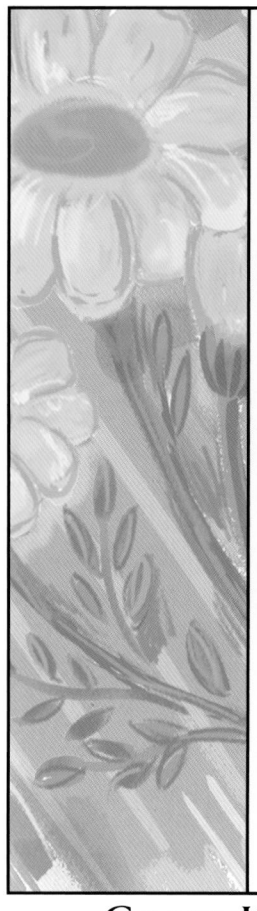

Making a

SLEEPYTIME PILLOW

For centuries folk herbalists have prescribed herbal "dream" pillows to promote a good night's sleep. These tiny pillows, filled with dried herbs, are placed inside or under your regular pillow. You can buy herbal sleep pillows already made, but you'll have more fun—and your herbs will be fresher and last longer—if you make one yourself. Many herb stores and health food markets provide not only the dried herb ingredients, but also drawstring muslin bags that can be used as little pillows. (Do not use the drawstring; instead, stitch the top of the bag closed after putting the herbs in.) You can also use a large scarf or handkerchief or a small pillowcase folded up into roughly a 5-inch-by-5-inch square and then stitched around the edges; leave a 4-inch opening to insert the herbs.

For a wonderfully aromatic and sedating herb "stuffing," thoroughly mix together 1 heaping tablespoon each of lemon balm, hops, rose petals, lavender, and chamomile flowers. Spoon into your sleep pillow and sew the 4-inch opening closed. Flatten out lightly with your hands and place under your pillow or in the pillowcase.

GOTU KOLA
(*Centella asiatica*)

A native of marshy areas in many subtropical lands and the southern United States, the gotu kola plant has long been used therapeutically by Indian Ayurvedic practitioners and Chinese herbalists. In both cultures, gotu kola—also known as centella, marsh pennywort, sheep rot, and *brahmi* (in India)—is regarded as a powerful general tonic, much like ginseng, that promotes good health and longevity. In some subtropical countries, gotu kola is the traditional treatment for Hansen's disease (leprosy), a therapeutic use that has been investigated and endorsed by modern researchers. This medicinal action is due in large part to the plant's most powerful chemical constituent, asiaticoside, a potent antibacterial and immune stimulant that might have several other important therapeutic properties. The herb is also prescribed for psoriasis, phlebitis, and epilepsy and is used externally to promote healing and inhibit scarring.

Today, both Eastern and Western herbalists prescribe gotu kola most frequently as a general tonic and for insomnia (particularly chronic insomnia), anxiety, hyperactivity, and mental agitation. It is available as dried herb, powder, capsules, tea, and tincture.

Caution: Only take gotu kola under the care of a qualified practitioner and in commercially prepared formulations. Minor side effects may include skin rashes or headaches. If these occur, stop taking the herb and contact your practitioner. Large doses of the herb can have a dangerous narcotic effect. Do not use gotu kola if you are nursing or if you are using tranquilizers or sedatives. Older adults should start with the minimum dosage and increase it if necessary only on the advice of their practitioner.

O sleep, O gentle sleep!
Nature's soft nurse, how have I
frighted thee,
That thou no more wilt weigh my
eyelids down
And steep my senses
in forgetfulness?
—WILLIAM SHAKESPEARE,
HENRY IV

HOPS
(*Humulus lupulus*)

Famously known as an essential brewing ingredient of beer and ale, the dried flowers of the hops vine are also widely prescribed by herbalists for their sedating and sleep-promoting effects—a use that can be traced to ancient Rome. Back then, hops was commonly known as *lupus salictarius* (willow wolf) for its habit of wrapping itself tightly around willows and other trees. Used therapeutically throughout Europe since the eighth century, hops can also be eaten fresh in salads or steamed much like green vegetables.

Researchers have confirmed that hops, a member of the hemp (Cannabinaceae) family, is a central nervous system depressant that relaxes smooth muscle and relieves spasms. Hops is therefore often prescribed for indigestion, stomach cramps, and irritable bowel syndrome. The plant's sedating and sleep-inducing actions, however, are more well known and believed to be the re-

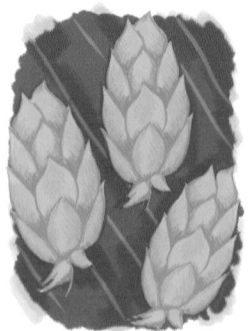

HOPS
(*Humulus lupulus*)

sult of the interaction of two of its main ingredients: the bitters humulon and lupulon, found in the female flowers or hop cones.

Taken internally, hops is available as dried herb (flowers or hop cones), tincture, capsules, and teas (usually in combination with other calming herbs). Follow your practitioner's or the manufacturer's directions.

Caution: Do not take hops if you have been diagnosed with depression. Its slightly narcotic effect may exacerbate some of your symptoms. There have been anecdotal reports—as yet unsubstantiated—suggesting that hops promotes menstruation. Err on the side of caution and do not take the herb if you suspect you are pregnant or you are trying to conceive. There has also been evidence, again anecdotal, that hops inhibits the sex drive. If you are experiencing impotence, diminished sex drive, or any sexual dysfunction, avoid taking hops until you consult with a qualified herbal practitioner.

I arise from dreams of thee
In the first sweet sleep of night,
When the winds are breathing low,
And the stars are shining bright.
—PERCY BYSSHE SHELLEY,
"THE INDIAN SERENADE"

SEDATING SCENTS

Inhaling the aroma of sleep-inducing essential oils is a lovely way to end the day. In a diffuser, combine 3 to 5 drops each of geranium, jasmine, lemon balm, Roman chamomile, and rose oils. Place the diffuser in your bedroom (on a fire-resistant plate, if you are using a diffuser with candles), and allow this subtly fragrant blend to sweep you off to dreamland.

LEMON BALM
(Melissa officinalis)

Lemon balm—also known as balm, honey-plant, melissa, and sweet balm—has a long history as both a nonmedicinal drink and a therapeutic tea. It is one of the mildest of the sedating herbs—with antispasmodic properties as well—and it is especially effective in gently relaxing the body and calming the emotions prior to sleep. A pungently lemon-scented member of the mint family, lemon balm was a favored daily toddy in sixteenth- and seventeenth-century England. But it is in modern Europe (Germany to be precise) that lemon balm has been most closely studied for its medicinal effects.

Therapeutically, lemon balm is a very close relative of chamomile: Both are mildly sedating, have antispasmodic action, and relieve indigestion. Lemon balm's sedating action, however, seems specifically to target brain activity, and it is frequently prescribed for insomnia and other sleep problems in which there is known depression, anxiety, stress, or hyperactivity. In Germany, in fact, it is the main ingredient of a popular medicine, *Melissengeist*, which is prescribed for just those symptoms.

Several ingredients in the plant's volatile oil, including citronellal, citral, and geraniol, all have central nervous system calming effects. They also act as antispasmodics and astringents.

Taken internally for insomnia, poor sleep, restlessness, excitability, headaches, depression, and heart palpitations, lemon balm is available as dried herb, tincture, tea, capsules, and oil. In Europe it is available in ointment form as a treatment for herpes simplex. In teas it is often combined with chamomile, valerian, and passionflower for a potent nighttime soporific.

Lemon balm is considered a very safe herb and it is often prescribed for children.

And all my days are trances,
And all my nightly dreams
Are where thy grey eye glances,
And where thy footstep gleams—
In what ethereal dances,
By what eternal streams.
—EDGAR ALLAN POE,
"TO ONE IN PARADISE"

PASSIONFLOWER
(Passiflora incarnata)

Gardeners prize this wonderfully aromatic subtropical vine for its beautiful, purple-ringed, peach and yellow flowers. Native to the southern United States and introduced into Europe in the late 1800s, the passion-flower plant also produces an edible, sweet-tasting yellow fruit. Its Latin and common names, which literally mean "flowers of the passion," refer to the resemblance of various parts of the plant to the instruments of death used during Christ's crucifixion.

Research studies have demonstrated that both the fruit—fresh or dried—and the whole flowering plant have strong sedating, hypnotic, antispasmodic, and pain-relieving properties. Passionflower also reduces high blood pressure. It is most frequently used for its ability to inhibit central nervous system activity and treat more extreme and pernicious forms of insomnia and disturbed sleep patterns that may be precipitated by chronic stress and accompanied by anxiety, rapid heartbeat, and excessive worry. Passionflower is also used to treat indigestion, pain, neuralgia, shingles, and Parkinson's disease and to relieve the symptoms of alcohol and drug withdrawal.

PASSIONFLOWER
(Passiflora incarnata)

Other Helpful Herbs to Promote Relaxation and Sleep

- ■ CHAMOMILE
- ■ CHASTE TREE
- ■ KAVA KAVA
- ■ LAVENDER
- ■ LIME BLOSSOMS
- ■ MINT
- ■ THYME
- ■ VALERIAN

Taken internally, passionflower is found in commercial homeopathic or herbal remedies and as dried or fresh leaves and fruit, capsules, tincture, and tea.

Caution: Passionflower is a strong sedative and hypnotic and should only be taken under the care of a qualified practitioner. Likewise, use only professionally prepared products and never harvest your own herb; another species of the plant, *Passiflora caerulea*, contains cyanide. Use low-strength preparations for adults over age 65.

Minor side effects include gastric upset and diarrhea. Discontinue use and call your practitioner if these occur. More serious side effects may include excessive sleepiness. Do not take passionflower during the day if you operate heavy machinery or drive. Use caution when combining with prescription sedatives.

Sharpening
Your Memory

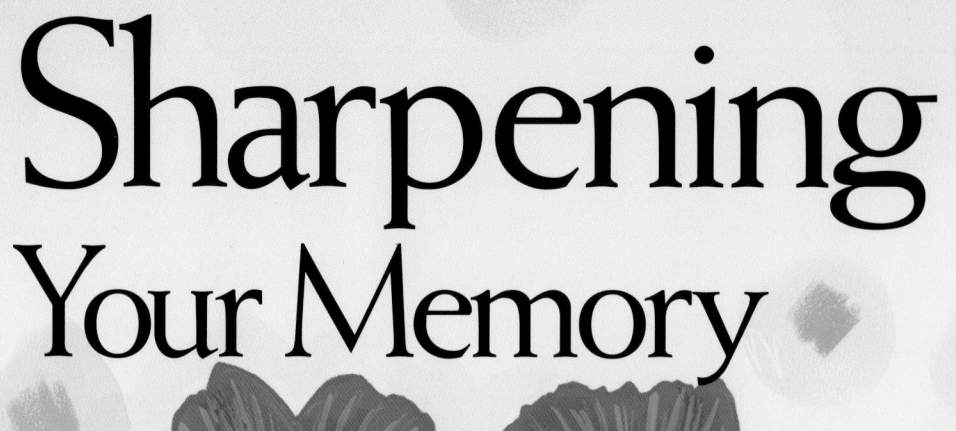

BRAIN. *An apparatus with*
which we think
that we think.
—AMBROSE BIERCE,
THE DEVIL'S DICTIONARY

MEMORIES . . .

It is normal to suffer temporary bouts of forgetfulness, confusion, lack of concentration, and just general "fuzziness." Overwork, stress, worry, poor diet, too much alcohol, too little sleep, and not enough exercise—along with certain ailments and medications—are all culprits in dulling the cerebral senses from time to time.

Chronic memory problems and persistent loss of mental acuity are often the results of a lifetime's accumulated damage to the circulatory and vascular systems. Poor blood circulation to the brain and heart, constricted or obstructed blood vessels, and oxygen-depleted blood all may contribute to the memory loss, confusion, and lack of clarity associated with aging and diseases such as senility, coronary artery disease, stroke, and Alzheimer's.

Select herbs act as circulatory and blood tonics. They are famed for their ability to dilate constricted arteries and veins, inhibit blood clotting, stimulate the circulatory system, increase blood circulation, and raise oxygen levels in the blood. The collective effect of such herbs is to increase the flow of oxygen-rich blood to the brain and thus enhance memory and mental functions. Here are five of the best brain-boosting herbs.

GINKGO
(Ginkgo biloba)

In recent years, ginkgo has garnered enormous scientific and popular attention for its therapeutic role in enhancing brain function, memory, reaction time, and alertness in people with Alzheimer's disease and other mild to moderate mental impairments.

Also known as maidenhair tree and silver apricot, ginkgo is native to China and Japan—where it is revered as a sacred, "living fossil," the origins of which can be traced back hundreds of millions of years to the Triassic period, when dinosaurs first appeared. Transplanted to Europe in the 1700s, gingko is now widely prescribed in both the East and the West for a variety of ailments, including colds, allergies, asthma, bedwetting, arthritis, vertigo, poor eyesight and poor hearing, vaginal infections, and premature ejaculation.

> *I have nothing to declare*
> *except my genius.*
> —OSCAR WILDE,
>
> *TO A CUSTOMS OFFICER UPON*
> *ARRIVING IN AMERICA IN 1882*

Ginkgo's greatest therapeutic property, however, is its clinically proven effectiveness against cerebral and circulatory problems. Two of the plant's major chemical ingredients—flavone glycosides and terpene lactones—act together to dilate blood vessels, prevent blood clotting, dramatically increase blood circulation to the brain and heart, and boost blood-oxygen levels. The increased flow of oxygen-rich blood to the brain and heart makes ginkgo a potent weapon against vascular diseases that involve constricted or obstructed blood vessels, poor blood circulation, and oxygen-depleted blood. Such diseases include coronary artery disease, stroke, diabetes, senility, and Alzheimer's, as well as associated

GINKGO
(*Ginkgo biloba*)

vascular problems such as poor memory, confusion, lack of concentration, and diminished mental acuity.

Both the nuts and leaves of the ginkgo plant have therapeutic properties, but the nuts (or "kernels") are rarely available commercially. Ginkgo leaves are widely available, however, in dry bulk, capsules, tea, and tinctures. You can also find ginkgo biloba extract in most health food stores. Herbalists recommend buying only professionally prepared, over-the-counter ginkgo products.

Caution: Minor side effects may include irritability, restlessness, diarrhea, headaches, and nausea. If any of these symptoms occur, consult your practitioner. Check with your practitioner before using ginkgo if you have a blood-clotting disorder, hemophilia, or are nursing. Always takes ginkgo at the smallest recommended dosages.

GINSENG (ASIAN)
(*Panax ginseng*)

All the ginsengs—among which Asian ginseng is the most potent and expensive—are adaptogenic herbs. These are herbs that promote optimal mental and physical health by increasing the body's resistance to physical, chemical, biological, and emotional stress. Simply put, the ginsengs are superb energy tonics, and Asian ginseng is the best. Frequently prescribed to enhance overall physical and mental well-being, Asian ginseng is especially renowned for increasing mental clarity, powers of concentration, and short-term memory.

One of the "superherbs"—together with angelica sinensis, echinacea, garlic, ginkgo, and St. John's wort—ginseng may be the most studied of all the herbal medicines. Besides being rich in several essential vitamins and minerals, many of Asian ginseng's active chemical ingredients have remarkable therapeutic effects. The ginsenosides strengthen the immune system, increase the body's ability to deal with fatigue and stress, and enhance learning. Panaxin is a cardiotonic that directly stimulates the circulatory and central nervous systems. Panoxic acid normalizes and stimulates the metabolism and helps lower cholesterol levels. Panaquilon nourishes and regulates the hormonal systems. Asian ginseng's essential oils appear to stimulate specific brain functions.

Asian ginseng is taken internally as a general tonic to enhance mental and physical well-being and performance; to improve memory, mental clarity, and concentration; to fight the effects of fatigue, stress, illness, and environmental pollutants; and to heal a damaged immune system. It is available as fresh, dried, or freeze-dried root, root powder, capsules, tablets, and prepared tea. It is frequently combined in herbal formulas with other tonifying herbs, such as ginkgo.

Caution: Use only under the direction of a qualified practitioner if you have asthma, a blood-clotting disorder, diabetes, emphysema, fibrocystic breasts, hay fever, heart disorder, or high blood pressure. Minor side effects may include headache, insomnia, anxiety, breast soreness, or skin rash. Serious side effects may include asthma attacks, increased blood pressure, heart palpitations, or postmenopausal uterine bleeding. If any of these symptoms occur, stop using Asian ginseng and consult your doctor.

I remember, I remember
The house where I was born,
The little window where the sun
Came peeping in at morn.
—THOMAS HOOD,
"I REMEMBER, I REMEMBER"

CHINESE FOXGLOVE ROOT
(*Rehmannia glutinosa*)

Another of Chinese herbal medicine's esteemed tonic herbs, Chinese foxglove root—or rehmannia, as it is more commonly called in both the East and West—has been prescribed by Asian herbalists for centuries as a stimulating blood tonic and a soothing "yin" tonic. (Yin is the cooling, moistening, and calming half of the yin-yang spiritual energy dynamic that permeates Chinese medicine, philosophy, and culture.)

Rehmannia has different therapeutic properties, depending on the part of the plant used and whether it is eaten cooked or raw. The cooked root is prescribed as a blood tonic that nourishes and strengthens bones, tendons, marrow, eyes, and ears. Rehmannia root is often steamed in wine to make a tonic specifically prescribed to inhibit the effects of aging, including memory loss and senility. The steamed tubers also nourish and tonify the blood and stimulate healthy blood circulation to the heart and brain. The raw tubers are prescribed as a yin tonic that nourishes and supports the kidneys and liver and acts to lower high blood pressure. Clinical studies confirm that rehmannia is a cardiotonic with blood-pressure-lowering properties.

Taken internally, raw or cooked, rehmannia is prescribed as a blood tonic, circulatory stimulant, hypotensive, and an antiaging treatment particularly effective against premature senility, premature graying of hair, memory loss, poor eyesight and poor hearing, and painful, stiff joints.

The prepared root and the raw version are available dried, and rehmannia is also available as raw root and tubers, decoctions, tonics, and wines. The herb is frequently found in many of traditional Chinese medicine's most famous herbal formulas, including Four Things Soups, the most esteemed and prescribed female tonic.

Caution: Talk to a qualified practitioner of Chinese herbal medicine about how and when to take rehmannia. Before taking it, consult with your practitioner if you have irritable bowel syndrome or other digestive problems; the cooked herb can cause abdominal distention and diarrhea.

I think, therefore I am.
—RENÉ DESCARTES,
DISCOURSE ON METHOD

I think I think; therefore,
I think I am.
—AMBROSE BIERCE,
THE DEVIL'S DICTIONARY

POLYGONUM/FO-TI
(*Polygonum multiflorum*)

For centuries Asian herbalists have prescribed polygonum—called *ho shou wu* in China—to inhibit and even reverse many of the effects of premature aging. Known in the West as fleeceflower root and marketed commercially as fo-ti, polygonum is China's premier "longevity herb," variously

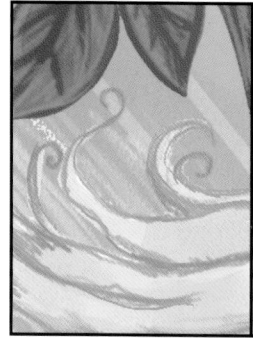

prescribed for poor memory, premature senility, gray hair, low sex drive, weak vision, impotence, wrinkles, and insomnia.

Now that it is increasingly popular in the West, herbalists prescribe polygonum as a stimulating tonic that nourishes the blood, liver, and kidneys; energizes the body; enhances brain and heart function; and slows down the aging process. Additionally, there is much anecdotal evidence that polygonum, taken over the long term, will return gray hair to its original color. Researchers have yet to confirm the hair-coloring properties of polygonum, but they have demonstrated in clinical studies that the herb is a cardiotonic with vasodilating, anticoagulant, hypotensive, anti-inflammatory, and antitumor actions.

Polygonum's combined anticoagulant and vasodilating actions inhibit blood clotting and increase blood flow to the brain and heart. Enhanced blood flow to the brain can help prevent short-term memory loss and inability to concentrate.

Polygonum is most frequently taken internally for its cardiotonic, blood tonifying, and antiaging effects. It is available in Asian pharmacies and herbal stores, as well as many commercial health stores, as dried root, decoctions, tincture, tonics, tonic wines, and capsules. It is frequently combined with similarly acting tonic herbs, such as ginseng and Chinese foxglove root.

Caution: Mild side effects may include flushing, diarrhea, and gastrointestinal upset. In Asian herbal medicine, the herb is contraindicated for people with diarrhea or chest congestion. Some traditional Chinese medicine sources also advise that polygonum not be taken with onions, chives, or garlic.

ROSEMARY
(*Rosmarinus officinalis*)

The aromatic rosemary plant—once known as "rose of the sea" and "sea mist"—is steeped in lore. Long a symbol of love, friendship, and loyalty, it has been worn by brides to demonstrate their fidelity and carried by funeral attendees to ward off demons. Its medicinal use, going back thousands of years, is equally colorful. In ancient Greece, philosophers and students wore rosemary garlands—or *coronariums* (the plant's Old Latin name)—to stimulate the brain and improve memory. The ancient Romans—who used it extensively in their cuisine—brought it to Britain, where it was variously prescribed to prevent aging, wrinkles, rotting teeth, and coughs. Shakespeare immortalized the plant in this famous line from *Hamlet*, "There's Rosemary, that's for Remembrance," a reference to the herb's memory-boosting powers. And by the seventeenth century, the famous herbalist Nicholas Culpeper was recommending rosemary to treat "dullness of the mind and senses."

As is often the case with herbal fact and fiction, much of the legend around rosemary has a basis in fact. Modern herbalists frequently prescribe rosemary as a circulatory and central nervous system stimulant. Researchers confirm that the leaves and oil of the plant contain a chemical ingredient called borneol that is believed to increase blood flow at the surface of the skin and generally stimulate the circulatory system, acting primarily as a vasodilator and thereby increasing blood flow to the heart and brain. When the brain receives more oxygen-rich blood, cerebral functioning—including memory and concentration—is enhanced.

This very remarkable man
Commends a most practical plan:
You can do what you want
If you don't think you can't,
So don't think you can't
think you can.
—CHARLES INGE,
ON MONSIEUR COUÉ

Rosemary also has antispasmodic, antibacterial, antifungal, and some pain-relieving properties. Besides its stimulating and vasodilating properties, rosemary is also prescribed for internal use as a digestive aid, decongestant, muscle relaxant, tension reducer, and antidepressant. Externally, it is used to treat skin infections and fungi.

Rosemary is available as dried herb, tincture, tea, and two types of oil—one for internal use and the other for external application.

Caution: Consult with your practitioner before taking rosemary oil internally, and always take rosemary—in any form—at prescribed dosages. Even in small doses, the oil may cause mild gastric and intestinal upset. Taken in large amounts, rosemary oil can be poisonous. Do not confuse the rosemary used internally with the oil that is applied topically. Never ingest the latter.

More Helpful Advice
YOU'VE GOTTA HAVE "HUP"

Huperzine A, that is—or HupA, for short—the newest and potentially most exciting herbal supplement to join the arsenal of herbs and drugs that treat the memory loss, mental impairment, and dementia that characterize Alzheimer's disease (AD). A naturally occurring compound found in Chinese club moss (*Huperzia serrata*), traditional Chinese medicine practitioners have long prescribed club moss (or *Qian Ceng Ta*) for fevers, inflammations, bleeding, bruises, and hemorrhoids. Then several years ago, Chinese researchers discovered that the herb contained an alkaloid, huperzine A, which had many of the same therapeutic actions—but none of the side effects or liver toxicity—as tacrine and donepezil, the prescription drugs used to treat AD. Further studies by Chinese and American researchers demonstrated that HupA not only successfully treated memory loss, dementia, and impaired cognitive function—in animal and human subjects—but that it also appeared to act as a preventive against the degenerative brain damage associated with aging. Talk to your practitioner about whether HupA—in commercially prepared extracts—is right for you or a loved one.

Fighting
the Blues

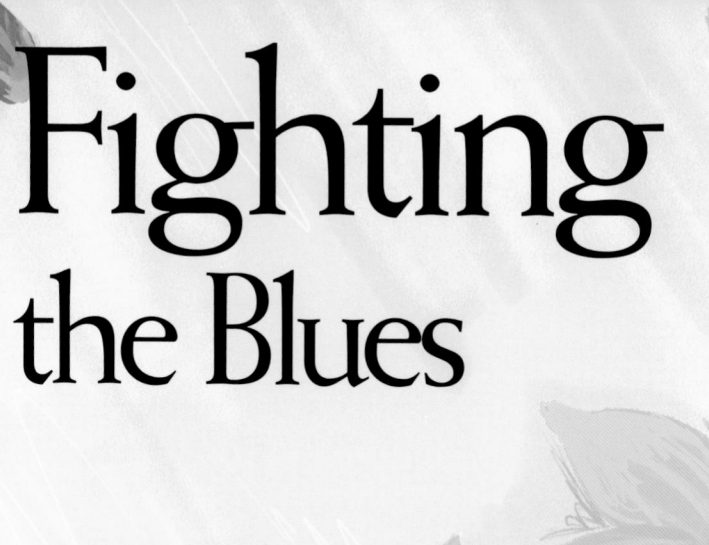

*Sadness flies on the wings
of the morning,
and out of the heart of
darkness comes the light.*
—JEAN GIRAUDOUX

THE HERBAL WAY TO TREAT MILD DEPRESSION AND SEASONAL AFFECTIVE DISORDER (SAD)

However distressing and disruptive it may be, feeling depressed for a few days, or even a week or two, is often normal. We work and play at a fevered pitch, delicately balancing work, home, children, spouses, bosses, relatives, and neighbors. We suffer temporary losses, minor illnesses, changes of jobs, fractious coworkers, sassy teens, and road-raging motorists. We bend under the burdens of relentless stress, horrifying headlines, and our own unrealistic expectations. There are going to be times when we feel overwhelmed, anxious, melancholy, and exhausted; when we overeat or undereat, are unable to cope, or cannot get a good night's sleep.

Then, almost magically, we see daylight again, the shadows lift, we scoot out from under our temporary malaise, and we get back to the business of living. Most of us do, anyway. But when depressed symptoms go on for longer than a week or two, when we begin to feel helpless and hopeless, and when panic and anxiety prevent us from living wholly and happily, we may be clinically depressed. And we definitely need help, because depression kills more than 30,000 people a year.

This is a serious illness that frequently goes undiagnosed and untreated. Yet at least 18 million people in the United States alone struggle with some form of depression each year. If you have been experiencing two or more of the symptoms described in the first paragraph for more than two weeks, please see a qualified practitioner. If you are depressed, there are many treatments and combinations of treatments that can help the healing process immeasurably. Talk to your doctor or alternative practitioner right away.

Many herbs—both those described here and in Chapter 8, "Soothing the Spirit"—have been used with great success to supplement conventional treatments of depression. One herb in particular—St. John's wort—has emerged to stand on its own as a natural, safe antidepressant for mild to moderate cases of depression. It is a bona fide natural alternative to conventional antidepressants.

St. John's wort is also an effective treatment for the significant number of light-sensitive people who experience Seasonal Affective Disorder (SAD), a form of temporary depression that is cyclical in nature, occurs most frequently during the winter months, and is related to diminished sunlight. Peo-

Take a Walk
ON THE WILD SIDE

No, you can't walk off depression the way you walk off five extra pounds. No matter the pace or the passing scenery, depression takes time and therapy to heal. But a half-hour walk—preferably in nature, along a country road or park lane, but even just in new environs—can do much to ease the symptoms of depression. As our focus shifts from inner turmoil to the world around us, worries and fears retreat for a while. As we stride, our breathing becomes longer and deeper, sending more oxygen-rich blood to our hearts, brain, and muscles; anxiety and stress recede, clarity returns, aches and pains and palpitations disappear. We return to our homes or our work refreshed and revitalized.

ple with SAD have many of the same symptoms described earlier, but because SAD is time-limited, usually lasting only from late November to March, prescription drugs are often not the best choice for treatment. Light therapy with full-spectrum bulbs that mimic sunlight has been the preferred way to treat SAD. Several studies, however, strongly indicate that St. John's wort is an effective treatment for SAD, especially because it can be effective on a short-term basis, has relatively few side effects, and can be stopped without a long weaning process—often necessary with prescription drugs.

Again, we don't recommend either self-diagnosing or self-treating depres-

sion. If you suspect you are clinically depressed, work with a professional. But by all means, explore the possibility of using herbs as supplemental therapy; and in the case of St. John's wort, consider using it as an alternative to conventional drugs.

BALMONY
(Chelone glabra)

More commonly known as turtlehead or white turtlehead (*chelone* is from the Greek for "tortoise") because its small, white flowers resemble a tortoise's head, balmony has a long history of use among Native Americans and folk herbalists, though to date it has received little scientific attention. A beautiful perennial that inhabits North American swamps, balmony has been used as a digestive aid, a stimulating tonic for the whole body, and a normalizing and detoxifying tonic for the liver. Balmony's energizing actions no doubt led to its traditional use by Native Americans as an antidepressant and appetite stimulant. (Lethargy and eating disorders often characterize depression.)

Balmony's actions as a liver tonic may also contribute to the herb's antidepressant properties. Practitioners of traditional Chinese medicine (TCM) would certainly think so: Most view depression as a fundamental "energy" imbalance directly caused by poor liver function and stagnant *qi* (pronounced chee)—the fundamental life force (energy) that circulates throughout the body. For depression, traditional Asian herbalists therefore prescribe tonic herbs that act as general stimulants, normalize liver function, and promote the circulation of *qi*, or energy. Besides balmony, such herbs would include angelica sinensis, peony, and licorice, among others.

In the West, homeopaths also use a tincture made from balmony leaves to treat poor liver function, and herbalists prescribe the dried flower and leaves in tea form as a general tonic, liver tonic, appetite stimulant, digestive aid, and laxative. Available as dried herb, balmony's general energizing effects may make it a good supplemental herb in the treatment of mild depression, particularly where anorexia is a component of the depression. The tea is quite bitter, however, and is often mixed with other herbs to mask its taste.

Caution: No appreciable side effects are associated with balmony, but because this is a little-studied herb, consult a qualified herbal practitioner about whether balmony is a good supplemental herb for your condition.

Of Special Note: Practitioners of TCM also view obesity (see Chapter 13, "Losing Weight") as a problem of poor liver function and stagnant *qi*, and many of the same herbs recommended for treating depression in TCM are used to promote weight loss.

Life is real! Life is earnest!
And the grave is not its goal;
Dust thou art, to dust returnest,
Was not spoken of the soul.
—HENRY WADSWORTH
LONGFELLOW,
"A PSALM OF LIFE"

BASIL
(Ocimum basilicum)

The distinctly sweet and pungent-smelling *Ocimum basilicum* plant is usually called sweet basil—to distinguish it from the many other species of wild and cultivated basils, each with its own distinctive look, taste, smell, and use. Its common name is derived from the Greek *basilikon*, meaning "king," an homage to the herb's revered status worldwide.

One of the most famous of the culinary herbs, sweet basil also has been celebrated through the centuries for its diverse—and sometimes contradictory—mystical and

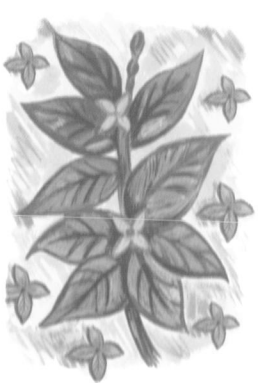

BASIL
(Ocimum basilicum)

medicinal effects. In Italy basil was used as a love potion, but in ancient Greece it was associated with terrible loss and bad luck. Percy Bysshe Shelley and John Keats immortalized basil as a symbol of love in separate poems, but the famous herbalist, Nicholas Culpeper, dismissed it with undisguised disgust as an abortifacient and aphrodisiac (it is neither). During the Middle Ages, basil was believed to be poisonous by some (they were wrong) and a spirit-lifting brain tonic by others (they were right). In the Middle East, basil was (and still is) planted on graves to soothe departed spirits and send them on their way.

It is also in the Middle East that basil leaves, eaten fresh or taken as a tea, are used daily by thousands to relieve depression and maintain good spirits. In fact, basil has a long history as an herbal treatment for "nervous" disorders and anxiety. Its essential oil, rich in estragol and eugenol, has both stimulating and mildly sedating actions and is an excellent antispasmodic. Available as dried and fresh herb, tea, and tincture, basil is most frequently prescribed to treat depression, anxiety, nervous headaches, migraines, and stomach cramps.

No appreciable side effects are associated with using basil.

> *I am the daughter of*
> *earth and water,*
> *And the nursling of the sky;*
> *I pass through the pores*
> *of the ocean and shores,*
> *I change, but I cannot die.*
> —PERCY BYSSHE SHELLEY,
> "TO A SKYLARK"

CLOVE
(*Syzygium aromaticum*)

The dried, dark-brown buds of the clove tree, commonly found on supermarket spice shelves and decorating holiday hams, contain aromatic essential oils that are rich in medicinal properties. First mentioned by ancient Chinese herbalists in the third century B.C. (to freshen one's breath before meeting the emperor), clove—like basil—acts as both a stimulant (to the circulatory system) and a sedative (to the nervous system). Therefore, it is a wonderful tonic for fatigue and general weakness, but also a very effective nervine for mild depression and anxiety. Clove is additionally prescribed for pain, nausea, colic, and bad breath.

Taken internally for nervous tension, stress, restlessness, anxiety, and insomnia, clove is available as dried buds, powdered buds, oil, decoction, capsules, and tea. Clove is most frequently prescribed as a tea, and there are commercially-prepared products available. To make your own antidepressant tea from clove buds, use a covered nonreactive pot to simmer 1/2 teaspoon of buds in 8 ounces of water for about 10 minutes. Drink plain or flavored with honey. For insomnia, gently simmer 1/2 teaspoon of buds in 8 ounces of milk for about 10 minutes, flavor with honey, and drink about 20 minutes before your bedtime. For mild depression, clove is frequently combined in teas with lime blossoms (linden), peppermint, and chamomile.

Caution: Mild stomach irritation may occur if clove is used in too high a dose or too frequently. Consult your practitioner before using clove if you have irritable bowel syndrome, ulcers, or other inflammatory stomach problems. Do not use clove oil internally. Although herbalists do prescribe the oil for internal use, the dosages are quite small and best administered by a qualified practitioner.

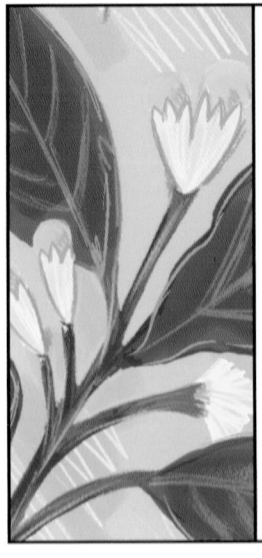

Bathing
YOUR BLUES AWAY

Soaking in a tubful of clove tea will ease anxiety, restlessness, frazzled nerves, tense and aching muscles—and prepare body and soul for a good night's sleep. Since you would need far too many tea bags to make a tub of clove tea, it is easier to prepare a large decoction from the buds beforehand. To do this, use a covered, nonreactive pan and simmer 1 to 1-1/2 teaspoons of whole clove buds in 3 quarts of water for about 25 minutes. Add the decoction to warm bath water and soak for at least 20 minutes.

There are two days in the week
about which and upon which
I never worry. Two carefree days,
kept sacredly free
from fear and apprehension.
One of these days is Yesterday. . . .
And the other day I do not worry
about is Tomorrow.
—ROBERT JONES BURDETTE,
THE GOLDEN DAY

ST. JOHN'S WORT
(*Hypericum perforatum*)

Also known as witch's herb, grace of God, and pennyjohn, the June-blooming, yellow-flowered St. John's wort plant has a long and celebrated herbal history as a wound-healer and infection fighter. From ancient Greek and Roman times, right up through the Middle Ages, herbalists used the plant almost exclusively for these two therapeutic properties. Like many herbs, St. John's wort was also endowed with mystical powers, and its flowers and leaves were used as talismans against demons, evil, and misfortune, and as offerings to the gods for bountiful harvests. (The plant blooms in late June, at the start of the traditional planting season.)

During the Middle Ages, St. John's wort also emerged as a treatment for "hysteria" and "madness," applications discovered, perhaps, when infusions of the herb were given to unfortunate souls "possessed by demons." In fact, the medieval exorcists who used St. John's wort for such purposes were on the right track. Today, St. John's wort (also commonly called hypericum) is considered by many to be the best herbal treatment for mild to moderate depression and SAD. It is also the subject of intense scientific research for its antiviral, antibacterial, and antitumor properties.

Researchers worldwide have confirmed that hypericin and pseudohypericin, two primary ingredients of St. John's wort, appear to significantly reduce or eliminate many of the symptoms of SAD and mild to moderate depression, including melancholy, depressed feelings, low energy, fa-

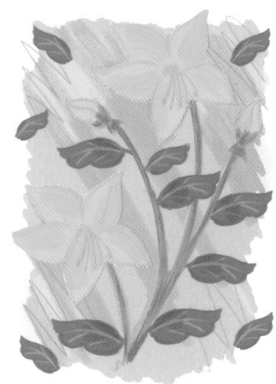

ST. JOHN'S WORT
(Hypericum perforatum)

tigue or exhaustion, irritability, poor concentration, anxiety, panic attacks, sleep disturbances, and eating disorders. Just as impressive as its depression-fighting properties are the relatively few side effects associated with using St. John's wort. Some prescription antidepressants, on the other hand, although indispensable for severe depression, are notorious for a wide range of unpleasant to dangerous side effects.

Taken internally as an antidepressant and to treat SAD, insomnia, anxiety, and eating disorders, St. John's wort is available as dried herb, tincture, tea, oil, and capsules. To treat depression, St. John's wort is frequently prescribed in capsule form—300 mg taken three times a day. For maximum effectiveness, all St. John's wort (or hypericum) products should be standardized to contain a minimum of 0.3 percent hypericin, the herb's most active antidepressant component.

Caution: Do not self-diagnose or self-treat depression or mood disorders. Depression is a serious illness, and any diagnosis and treatment plan should be made in consultation with a qualified practitioner.

Generally mild and transient side effects are associated with taking St. John's wort, including stomach upset and skin rashes. The most reported (and sometimes most exaggerated) side effect is photosensitivity (oversensitivity to the sun's skin-burning effects). At therapeutic doses—and with the use of sunscreens and cover-ups—this effect should not be a problem for most users. People who work outdoors, however, should consult with their practitioners about taking extra precautions if they use St. John's wort.

Emotion is the chief source of all becoming conscious. There can be no transforming of darkness into light and of apathy into movement without emotion.
—CARL JUNG, THE PRACTICE OF PSYCHOTHERAPY

Other Helpful Herbs:

For relieving the anxiety, restlessness, heart palpitations, irritability, and insomnia that may accompany mild depression and SAD, try using
- black cohosh,
- chamomile,
- kava kava,
- lavender, skullcap,
- and/or valerian.

See Chapter 8, "Soothing the Spirit," for more information about calming and sedating herbs.

A Cautionary
Note About
ST. JOHN'S WORT:

Early research indicated that St. John's wort had therapeutic properties similar to those of a group of antidepressant drugs called
monoamine oxidase inhibitors (MAOIs), among which Nardil and
Parnate are the most well-known. MAOIs may precipitate potentially
deadly side effects when combined with food, beverages, or drugs
that contain the amino acids tyramine and monoamine. People taking
St. John's wort, therefore, were often warned against consuming such
products, including red wine, sharp cheeses, pickled and smoked
meats and fish, soy products, raisins, bananas, decongestants, and
certain allergy medications.

Later studies, however, suggested that St. John's wort had minimal MAOI effects and instead was similar in action to Prozac—a safer,
non-MAOI prescription antidepressant. In fact, the therapeutic actions of St. John's wort appear similar to those of at least three different kinds of conventional antidepressants. And to date, no definitive
conclusions have been reached about just how it works. Err on the
side of caution and talk to your practitioner about whether you
should avoid certain foods, drinks, and medications if you take St.
John's wort.

Losing
Weight

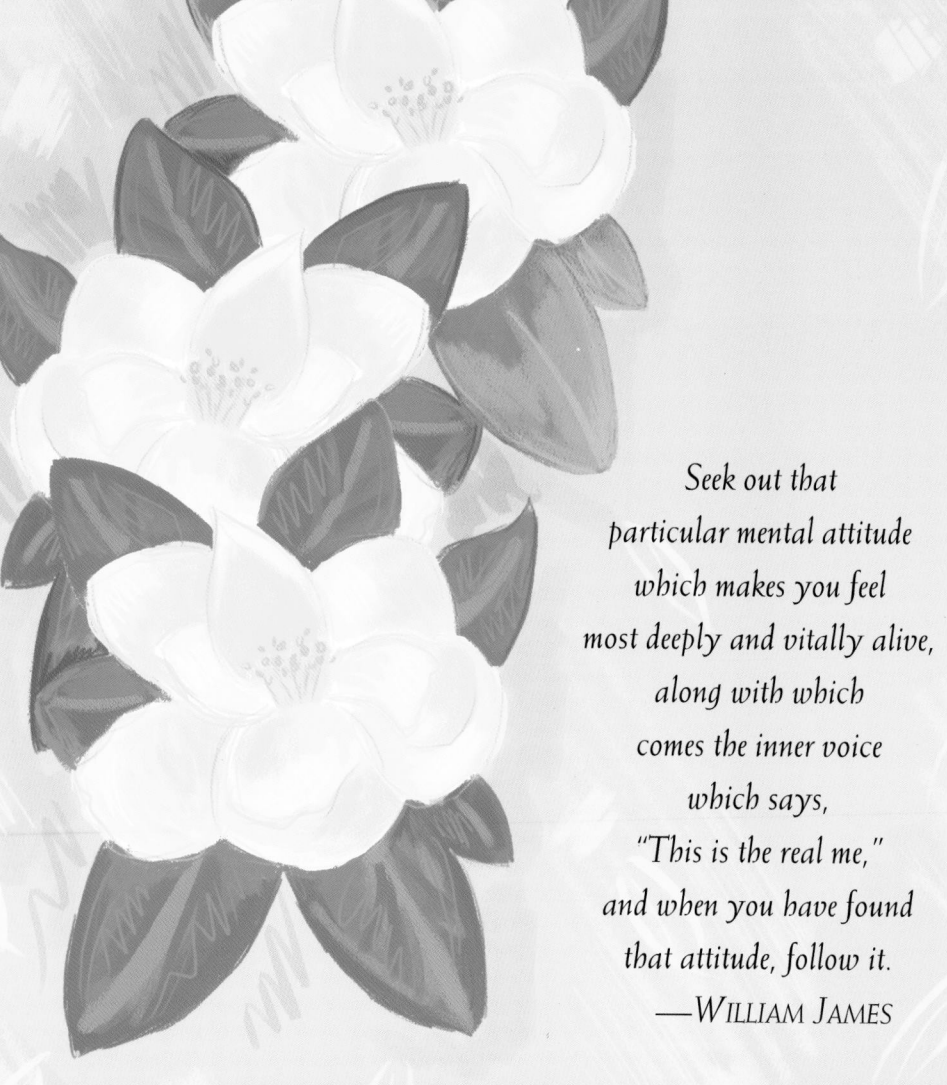

*Seek out that
particular mental attitude
which makes you feel
most deeply and vitally alive,
along with which
comes the inner voice
which says,
"This is the real me,"
and when you have found
that attitude, follow it.*
—WILLIAM JAMES

HERBAL REMEDIES TO PROMOTE WEIGHT LOSS AND CONTROL THE APPETITE

There is no magic bullet for losing weight—certainly no safe one. If you want to shed pounds safely and keep them off, there is only one way to go: Eat less and exercise more, a day at a time, for the rest of your life.

Most of us know when we are overweight—that is, 20 pounds or more over the recommended weight for our gender, height, and body frame. It's not just a matter of our favorite clothes no longer fitting us. When we are overweight, we feel sluggish, bloated, and easily winded after exertion. We tire more quickly and have low energy levels. Despite the fact that we eat too much, we often have poor appetites and irregular eating habits. We frequently suffer bouts of indigestion, abdominal bloating, water-weight gain, diarrhea, and/or constipation. Our internal organs—strained both by extra poundage and nutritionless, fatty, sugary foods—cannot function optimally when we are overweight. This is especially true of the liver, kidneys, spleen, and pancreas—responsible for detoxifying the blood, breaking down and eliminating wastes, and regulating blood and sugar levels. But it is often the intricate coronary artery system, and the heart at its center, that take the worst beating from fatty diets and lack of exercise.

Of course, our self-esteem suffers terribly, too, when we are overweight. But it is our health that is truly held hostage by obesity. And at the absolute worst end of the health spectrum, being chronically overweight makes us prime candidates for heart disease, high blood pressure, heart attack, stroke, diabetes, some cancers, and early death.

Certainly there are herbs that can suppress the appetite—chickweed, dandelion, vervain, and yerba maté, to name a few. And kelp—a regulator of the thyroid gland—is a favorite ingredient in many herbal weight-loss formulas (where it is often called laminaria). But suppressing the appetite on a short-term basis produces only short-term results—as anyone who has been caught on the "diet pill–weight loss –weight gain" pendulum can attest to.

Getting back to a healthy weight—and staying there—requires major lifestyle changes regarding diet and exercise. Getting our weight under control also requires that we strengthen and nourish the organ systems in our body that have been overtaxed by excess weight, inadequate nutrition, and fatty, toxic foods. When the latter

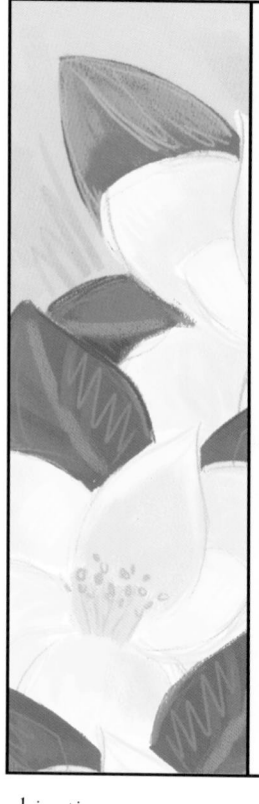

Maintaining Weight Loss

FOR A LIFETIME

If you want to maintain your weight for the long term, eat a low-fat diet, watch your intake of calories and sugar, get at least 30 minutes of aerobic (heart-pumping) exercise five times a week, and do 30 minutes of strength training (muscle-pumping) exercise at least three times weekly—strong muscles help accelerate and maintain weight loss. Start slowly, but do start. Day by day, incorporate one of these healthy habits into your daily routine. Working with a support group or a partner will make the changes feel less like drudgery and more like self-affirmation—which they are. Tell yourself you want to be here for the duration. You deserve to be strong, healthy, and happy.

objectives are part of a weight-loss program, there are indeed a number of herbs—many of which are classic "energy tonics"—that will provide excellent therapeutic support. Energy tonics can stimulate the metabolism, help in the excretion of excess fluids and wastes, stabilize the appetite, normalize digestion, and nourish and strengthen critical organs like the liver and kidneys so they can operate at optimal efficiency. The greatest herbal energy tonics are staple herbs of traditional Chinese medicine (TCM), but they are increasingly prescribed and available in the West. The following are a few of the best.

All that we are is the result of what we have thought. The mind is everything. What we think, we become.
—BUDDHA

ATRACTYLODES
(Atractylodes alba, A. macrocephalae)

Known as *bai zhu shu* and *cang zhu* in traditional Chinese medicine (TCM), atractylodes (also called white atractylodes and atractylus), is the most frequently prescribed herb for weight loss in Chinese herbal medicine. A general energy tonic with mildly stimulating properties, atractylodes is especially effective in normalizing the digestive system and regulating the appetite. It is also an excellent diuretic and is often given to strengthen the body overall and the muscles in particular. Its diuretic properties and digestive- and appetite-regulating actions are believed to be the effects of four of the root's primary ingredients: atractylol, atractylone, eudesmol, and hensol. It is frequently combined with other energy tonics for specific weight-control conditions. To treat anorexia, where the aim is both to normalize the appetite and nourish and strengthen the body, atractylodes is combined with poria, licorice, and codonopsis (all discussed later) in soups or in decoction or capsule form. For general weight loss it is often combined with tangerine peel (discussed later) in capsule form. For obesity associated with overeating, the powdered root is combined with licorice root in soups, capsules, or decoctions to reduce the appetite.

Atractylodes is available as powdered root, decoction, tea, soup, and capsules. Consult a qualified practitioner or herbalist who specializes in traditional Chinese medicine for advice on taking atractylodes.

Caution: No appreciable side effects are associated with atractylodes, but its use should be avoided in the presence of fever, excessive sweating, and dehydration.

CODONOPSIS
(*Codonopsis pilosulae*)

Commonly known as *dang shen*, codonopsis is extensively used in traditional Chinese medicine. However, it is rarely mentioned in the Western herbals, despite the fact that most of the major herbs used in Chinese medicine—and codonopsis is one of the best—are now available in herb stores,

Asian markets and pharmacies, and by mail order. Codonopsis is one of the most esteemed *qi* (pronounced chee) or energy tonics (along with astragalus, Asian ginseng, poria, and Chinese licorice, to name just a few), and it is often substituted for ginseng because it has many of the same therapeutic actions but delivers them less potently and more gently.

Herbalists prescribe codonopsis as an energy tonic to stimulate and regulate a poorly functioning metabolism characterized by fatigue, weakness, poor appetite, low energy, and bloating. If obesity or excessive weight gain is accompanied by breathlessness on mild exertion, heart palpitations, loose stools, digestive problems, and a lack of energy, codonopsis may increase metabolism, restore vitality, promote strength and endurance, aid in the excretion of excess fluids and waste materials, and promote more healthy eating patterns.

Codonopsis is available as dried or fresh root, tea, decoction, and capsules. Consult a qualified practitioner or herbalist who specializes in traditional Chinese medicine for advice on taking codonopsis.

No significant side effects or cautions are reported with the use of codonopsis.

Better to hunt in fields,
for health unbought,
Than fee the doctor
for a nauseous draught.
The wise, for cure,
on exercise depend;
God never made his work
for man to mend.
—JOHN DRYDEN

LICORICE
(Glycyrrhiza glabra,
G. uralensis)

Licorice is one of the most commonly used medicinal herbs in the West and the most frequently prescribed herb in the East. There it is called the "grandfather of Chinese herbs" and can be found in almost every major traditional Chinese formula. *Glycyrrhiza glabra* is most commonly used in the West, whereas *Glycyrrhiza uralensis* is used in Chinese medicine. Both varieties, however, have similar uses and properties, although *Glycyrrhiza uralensis*, or Chinese licorice, is believed to cause fewer side effects than the Western version that is associated with jitteriness and increased blood pressure when used excessively.

Licorice root is often used in combination herbal formulas because its sweet flavor masks the bitterness of many medicinal herbs, and it is considered a great "harmonizing" agent, helping the other herbs to work together more efficiently. On its own, however, and in moderation, licorice is itself an excellent stimulating tonic that raises energy levels, detoxifies the blood, strengthens the kidneys and spleen, and aids digestion. (It is also prescribed for coughs, diarrhea, and stomach ulcers.) Additionally, Chinese licorice is famous both for regulating blood sugar levels (it acts like an adrenal cortex hormone) and for treating anorexia. Herbalists from the Chinese tradition prescribe Chinese licorice tea as a daily restorative tonic. For weight loss, combined with equal parts atractylodes, codonopsis, and poria, Chinese licorice regulates the appetite, normalizes metabolism, raises energy levels, and relieves weakness and fatigue.

Licorice is available in a wide variety of forms, alone and in combination with other herbs, but is most frequently sold as dried root, decoction, liquid extract, tea, syrup, or capsules.

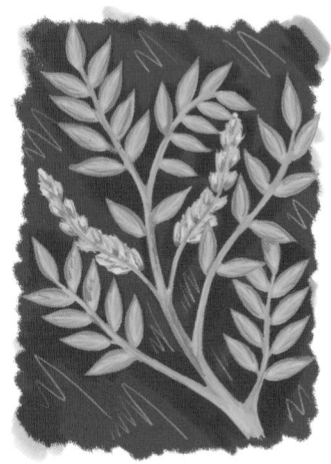

LICORICE
(Glycyrrhiza glabra,
G. uralensis)

Caution: Do not use licorice root if you have edema (water retention), high blood pressure, kidney disease, or glaucoma. Large amounts of licorice taken over a long period may also precipitate high blood pressure and edema. Take only in moderation and only under the advice and care of a qualified practitioner or herbalist.

i have noticed that when chickens quit quarreling over their food they often find that there is enough for all of them. i wonder if it might not be the same with the human race.
—DONALD ROBERT PERRY MARQUIS, ARCHY'S LIFE OF MEHITABEL, RANDOM THOUGHTS BY ARCHY

MAGNOLIA
(Magnolia officinalis, M. liliflora, M. grandiflora, M. virginiana)

Known in the West as sweetbay magnolia, swamp sassafras, and *flor de corazon* ("heart flower"); and in the East as *hsin-i, hou po,* and *xin yi hua,* the beautiful and sweet-smelling magnolia tree—emblematic of the American South—has a long history in Western and Chinese herbal medicine as a minor energy tonic.

The flowers and the bark have somewhat different therapeutic properties. Magnolia flower tea is often prescribed for its diuretic properties and to strengthen and stimulate the heart. (It is also used to treat sinus infection, congestion, and headaches.) The tea made from magnolia bark is used to stimulate the metabolism, relieve abdominal bloating and other stomach complaints, aid and normalize digestion, and improve mental clarity. Chinese herbalists additionally believe that a tea made from magnolia buds restores and stimulates energy throughout the body, reduces bloating, and helps eliminate excess fluids and wastes. Like poria, magnolia may be a useful weight-loss supplement—alone or in combination with other tonic herbs—for obesity accompanied by stress, low energy, high blood pressure, water retention, abdominal bloating, indigestion, and constipation.

The flowers and bark are available as dried herb, decoction, extract, and tea. Consult a qualified practitioner or herbalist about whether magnolia is right for you.

Caution: No appreciable side effects are associated with moderate magnolia use, but the herb should be avoided in the presence of fever, excessive sweating, and dehydration.

Imprisoned in every fat man a thin one is wildly signaling to be let out.
—CYRIL VERNON CONNOLLY,
THE UNQUIET GRAVE

PINELLIA
(Pinellia ternatae)

In Chinese herbal medicine, where it is known as *ban xia,* pinellia is used to treat all conditions in which there are excess fluids or mucous (what Asian herbalists call "dampness")—congestion, diarrhea, vomiting, and water retention. The root of the plant also acts as a mild tonic and diuretic and is prescribed to stimulate the metabolism, relieve fatigue, and aid digestion. It is a primary ingredient in two famous traditional Chinese herbal formulas frequently prescribed for obesity—Citrus and Pinellia (a combination of pinellia, poria, tangerine peel, licorice, and ginger) and Major Six Herbs (a combination of pinellia, poria, codonopsis, atractylodes, tangerine peel, licorice, ginger, and ziziphus).

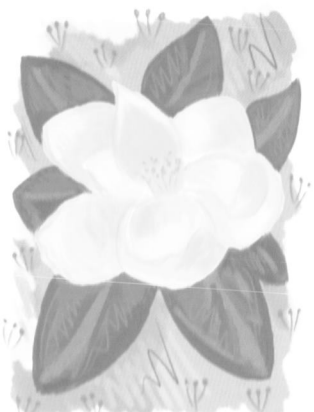

MAGNOLIA
(Magnolia officinalis, M. liliflora, M. grandiflora, M. virginiana)

Where poor metabolism, poor nutrition, abdominal bloating, and excessive overeating accompany obesity, Citrus and Pinellia is often prescribed. Where obesity is characterized by fatigue and breathlessness on exertion, heart palpitations, water retention, indigestion, and diarrhea, Major Six Herbs is frequently prescribed. With its mild, but effective energizing and diuretic effects, pinellia makes a fine supplemental herb in any weight-loss regimen.

Pinellia is available as dried and powdered bark, decoction, extract, and tea, and it is found in many Chinese patent herbal formulas. Consult a qualified practitioner or herbalist who specializes in traditional Chinese medicine for advice on taking pinellia.

Caution: No significant side effects are associated with the use of pinellia, but the herb should not be taken when there is dehydration.

PORIA/FU LING
(*Poria cocos*)

The North American mushroom—a cousin of similar varieties around the world—is also known as Indian bread in the West and as *fuk ling* and *hoelin* in the East. Poria is rarely used in the West anymore, even though it is one of the finest and gentlest of diuretics, and an excellent tonic with mild sedating properties. In Asia, however, it is the second most frequently prescribed of medicinal herbs (licorice is first). It is also an essential ingredient in the majority of the most famous traditional Chinese herbal formulas.

A superb energy and blood tonic that stimulates metabolism and restores general vitality, poria also tonifies and normalizes spleen, kidney, and bladder function and is a fine diuretic. It promotes good digestion, lowers blood pressure, and has sedating

effects. Poria—alone or in combination with other tonic herbs—is therefore an excellent choice for treating obesity accompanied by anxiety or stress, where there is high blood pressure, general debilitation, poor metabolism, abdominal bloating or fullness, water retention, indigestion, and constipation.

Poria, a fungus most often found clinging to tree roots, is available as dried, sliced herb, powdered herb, and capsules. Poria is also found in many of the most frequently prescribed Chinese herbal formulas. Consult a qualified practitioner or herbalist who specializes in Asian medicine for how and when to take the herb.

Caution: No appreciable side effects are associated with poria, but the herb should not be used when there is excessive urination.

Long have I loved what I behold.
The night that calms,
the day that cheers;
The common growth of
mother-earth Suffices me.
—*WILLIAM WORDSWORTH,*
PROLOGUE TO "PETER BELL"

TANGERINE PEEL/ CITRUS PEEL
(*Citrus reticulata*)

Known as *chen pi* in traditional Chinese medicine and sometimes called mandarin orange peel, aged tangerine or citrus peel is primarily prescribed to treat upset stomach and promote good digestion. However, it has a long history of use in treating obesity and is frequently combined with other "weight-loss" herbs, such as atractylodes (discussed earlier) for general weight loss where there is water retention, and pinellia (discussed earlier) for weight loss where there is poor metabolism, abdominal bloating, and overeating.

Taken internally as a general tonic for its stimulating and regulating effects, dried tangerine peel is especially useful for treating obesity where accompanied by low energy, sluggishness, abdominal bloating, indigestion, poor appetite, poor liver function, water retention, flatulence, and diarrhea. Tangerine or citrus peel is available at Asian food markets, Chinese pharmacies, and Western health food stores as aged dried peel, oil, tincture, tea, and capsules. It is also a common ingredient in herbal weight-loss formulas. Consult a qualified practitioner or herbalist who specializes in Asian medicine for advice on taking the herb.

Caution: No appreciable side effects are associated with the use of tangerine peel, but avoid its use if you have either a dry cough or a productive cough with excess phlegm.

The difference between perseverance and obstinacy is that one comes from a strong will, and the other from a strong won't.
—HENRY WARD BEECHER

Other Helpful Herbs:

- **FOR OBESITY ACCOMPANIED BY ABDOMINAL BLOATING AND WATER RETENTION: asparagus, calendula, dandelion, sarsaparilla, vervain**

- **FOR OBESITY ASSOCIATED WITH HYPOTHYROIDISM: kelp, turmeric**

- **FOR OBESITY ACCOMPANIED BY HIGH BLOOD PRESSURE AND CORONARY ARTERY DISEASE: astragalus, green tea, hawthorn**

- **FOR OBESITY CHARACTERIZED BY HIGH BLOOD CHOLESTEROL AND/OR POOR METABOLISM OF FATS: cleavers, gentian, ginger**

- **FOR OBESITY ACCOMPANIED BY ANXIETY, STRESS, AND DEPRESSION: St. John's wort**

Practicing
Natural Beauty

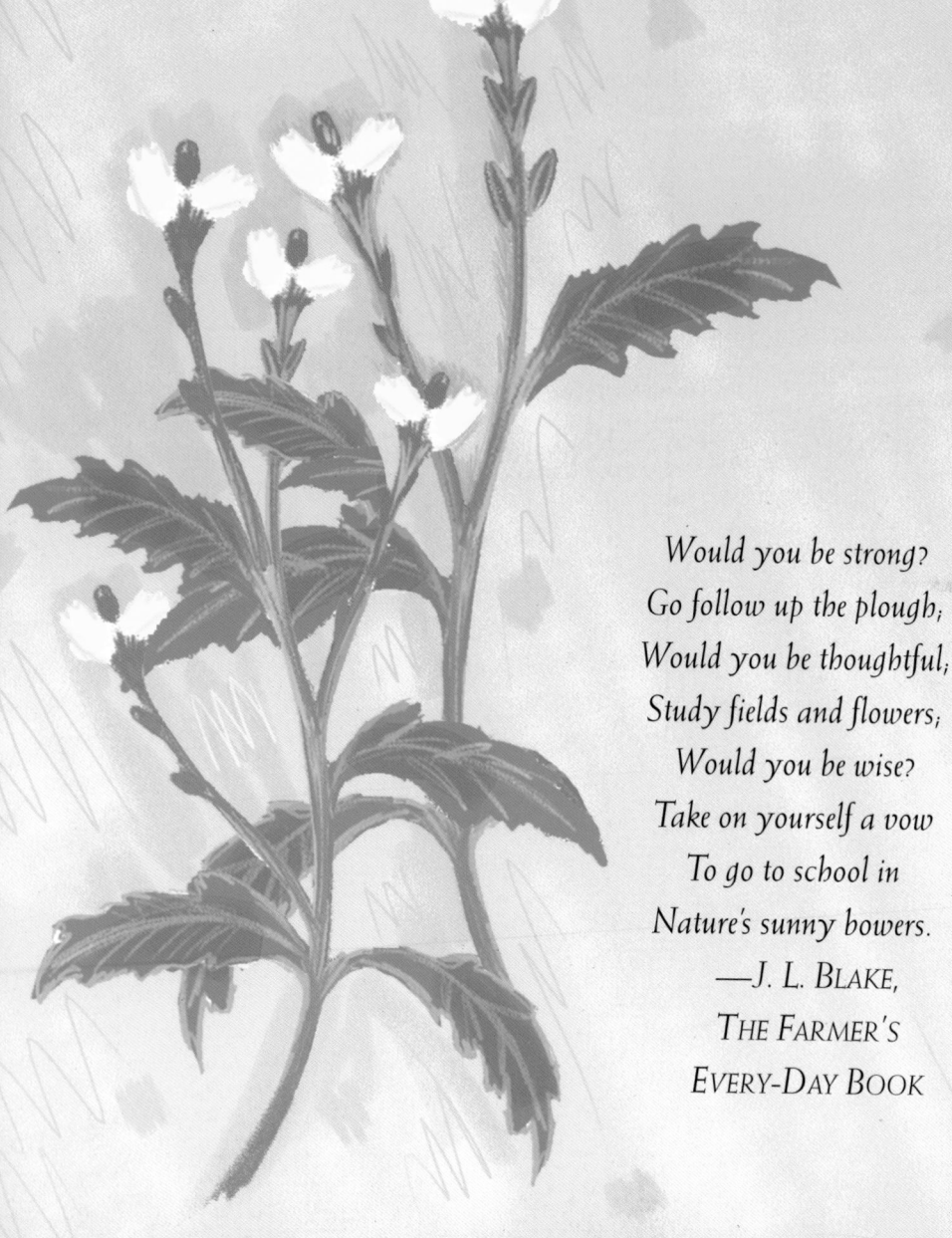

Would you be strong?
Go follow up the plough;
Would you be thoughtful;
Study fields and flowers;
Would you be wise?
Take on yourself a vow
To go to school in
Nature's sunny bowers.
—J. L. BLAKE,
THE FARMER'S
EVERY-DAY BOOK

NATURAL BEAUTY

Beauty, natural or not, is a subjective, relative state. What is beautiful in one culture, for example, is repugnant to another. What deliciously delights one person's fancy may leave another person dead cold. There are as many definitions of beauty as there are of love and art and nature and God and reality—of all, in fact, that is ultimately ineffable.

But we certainly can't feel beautiful—and real beauty is always in the heart of the beheld, not in the eyes of the beholder—if we don't feel healthy. Good health, then, is a fundamental fact of natural beauty. But what is good health? Again, health's a relative state. A chronically ill person who accepts herself, embraces life, laughs at nature's follies, and joyfully engages the world around her can exude a powerful beauty; yet another magnificently healthy individual who wraps himself in anger, self-doubt, and meanspiritedness may appear unwhole and diminished to the people around him.

The natural beauty that is founded on good health certainly includes eating fresh fruits, vegetables, and foods that are low in fat and sugars; supplementing our diets with vitamins, minerals, and other nutrients; drinking lots of water; getting regular exercise; managing our stress; and remembering to play. Natural beauty that is founded on good health also means putting aside our excesses: nicotine, alcohol, recreational drugs, fatty foods, too much TV, too little fresh air.

> *Go far, come near;*
> *You still must be*
> *The center of your own*
> *small mystery.*
> *—WALTER DE LA MARE,*
> *"GO FAR, COME NEAR"*

Many herbs have as long a history of cosmetic use as they do of medicinal use, but the herbs we feature here mainly deliver beauty from the inside out—as do most of the herbs in this book. When we nourish ourselves from the inside out, repairing what is broken in body and spirit, natural beauty always rises to the surface.

BARLEY
(Hordeum vulgare distochon)

Long used for its high nutritional value and soothing therapeutic properties, barley—or pearl barley, as it is often called—is a cereal crop traditionally served as a soup, stew, or in grain dishes. The water in which barley is soaked may be strained and used for a medicinal tea as well. Fields of barley's flaxen-colored, plaited-looking spikes nodding gently on slender grass stems are a familiar sight in America's Midwest, but barley grows in all temperate climates worldwide. It was the first cereal to be cultivated, and

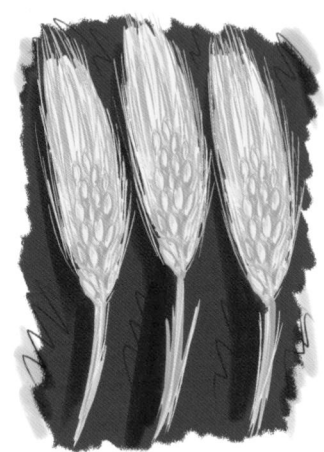

BARLEY
(Hordeum vulgare distochon)

its use stretches back to the Neolithic age. Ancient Egyptians believed it was a sacred gift from their revered goddess Isis, and they used it as a medicine, food, and fermented beverage similar to beer.

Frequently prescribed in folk medicine for irritable bowel syndrome, diarrhea, arthritis, rheumatism, and bronchitis, barley is additionally an excellent nutritional supplement and gentle tonic. Rich in proteins, vitamins B and E, complex carbohydrates, and soothing mucilage, barley is an especially good choice for those who are just beginning to explore the benefits of a healthy, whole grain-based diet. Barley breaks down slowly in the body and provides long-term energy and endurance. Its soothing properties make it a particularly beneficial nutritional supplement for people who have been ill or are simply run down. Barley also promotes good digestion and easy elimination of fluid and solid wastes, thereby supporting rich supplies of nourishing blood to the skin, muscles, and bones.

Barley—or pearl barley—is available in supermarkets and health food stores. Follow the preparation directions on the packaging.

Come forth into the light of things,
Let Nature be your teacher.
—WILLIAM WORDSWORTH,
"THE TABLES TURNED"

BILBERRY
(Vaccinium myrtillus)

Blueberry, hurtleberry, whortleberry, huckleberry—all are common names for the familiar, luscious-tasting blue fruits of the bilberry bush, a shrubby member of the heath (Ericaceae) family which is native to North America and northern Europe.

Most of us take our bilberries in jams, jellies, and pies—or fresh from the bush, preferably raw but occasionally covered in cream. The leaves and fruit of the bilberry bush, however, have a long history of medicinal use. Early Native Americans and English settlers used decoctions made from the roots and leaves to promote easy childbirths and to treat indigestion, urinary tract infec-

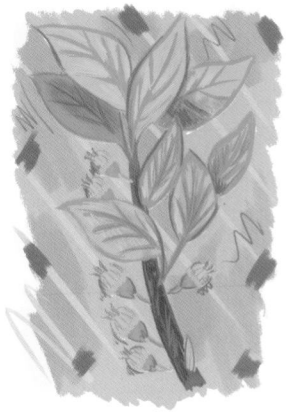

BILBERRY
(Vaccinium myrtillus)

tions, diarrhea, and inflammations. The North American Chippewa Indians burned dried bilberry flowers and inhaled their fumes to "cure" hysteria and madness. During the second World War, English pilots scheduled for night flights discovered that eating bilberry jam in the evening improved their night vision.

Bilberry tea, taken internally and made from fresh berries or bilberry tincture, is also prescribed by herbalists for gingivitis, mouth sores, varicose veins, and, most famously, for a range of eye disorders, including eye strain, poor night vision, cataracts, and glaucoma. Bilberry fruit is very high in vitamin C and contains a chemical ingredient called anthocyanoside; both components are believed responsible for the herb's therapeutic affect on vision.

Fresh bilberries or blueberries are available in supermarkets and produce stands. Dried berries, teas, and tinctures are available in health food stores and herb shops.

Caution: No side effects are associated with using bilberry fruit. However, a tea made from bilberry or blueberry leaves traditionally was used—and is still recommended by some herbalists—to control diabetes. A chemical found in the leaves,

neomyrtilicine, may moderate blood-sugar levels. However, the clinical evidence is scanty, and long-term use of bilberry-leaf tea can be toxic. Avoid tea made from bilberry leaves.

> *If you get simple beauty*
> *and nought else,*
> *You get about the best thing*
> *God invents.*
> —ROBERT BROWNING,
> "FRA LIPPO LIPPI"

EUCALYPTUS
(*Eucalyptus species*)

There are over 300 species of the eucalyptus tree whose uniquely smelling essential oil is familiar to most children and adults as Vicks VapoRub. Also known as Tasmanian blue gum and gum tree, eucalyptus oil has long been used by alternative and conventional medical practitioners as an external

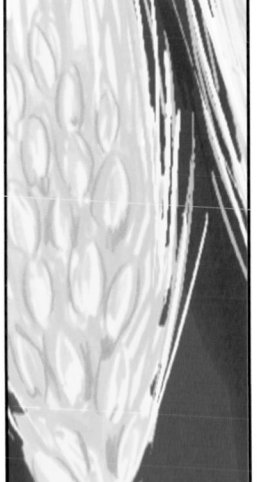

Barley and Blueberry

FOR BEAUTIFUL EYES

To brighten red, tired eyes and soothe eye strain, soak a clean white cotton cloth or compress in warm barley water (save the strained liquid used to cook the grains). Place over your eyes for 15 to 20 minutes. Drinking one to three cups a day of blueberry (bilberry) tea will also relieve eye strain—as well as night blindness, gingivitis, and canker sores!

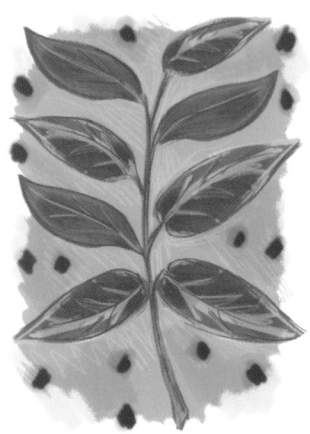

E U C A L Y P T U S
(Eucalyptus species)

treatment—in chest and throat rubs and steam vaporizers—for colds, sore throats, chest congestion, and bronchitis. While the plant's essential oil can be extracted from its roots, bark, and leaves, most eucalyptus products contain oil extracted from the leaves, which contain high concentrations of the plant's main medicinal ingredient, eucalyptol. Folk herbalists sometimes prescribe a diluted form of the oil to be taken internally, in small doses, for bronchitis and tuberculosis.

Give me a look, give me a face,
That makes simplicity a grace;
Robes loosely flowing, hair as free:
Such sweet neglect more taketh me
Than all th' adulteries of art;
They strike mine eyes,
but not my heart.
—BEN JOHNSON,
"EPICOENE, OR THE SILENT
WOMAN"

The external use of eucalyptus, however, is the most common mode of treatment, and it is not limited to relieving coughs and colds. Eucalyptus oil extracted from the leaves, and sometimes mixed with an emollient such as olive oil or almond oil, can soothe and heal dry, chapped skin. Mas-

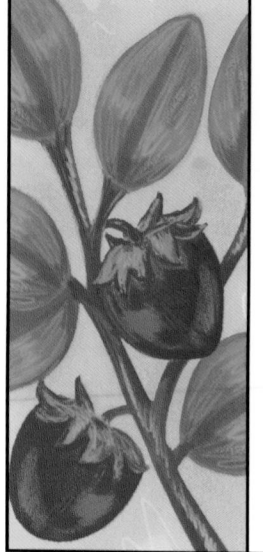

The Joys

OF JOJOBA

Jojoba *(Simmondsia chinensis)* has long been used by Native Americans as a topical treatment. Jojoba oil, extracted from the plant's seeds, is an excellent healer of dry, broken, chapped skin; chapped and blistered lips; dry, brittle hair; and dry, scaly scalp.

Many herbalists believe that regularly massaging the scalp with jojoba essential oil will result in new hair growth. You can find jojoba in many commercial and cosmetic preparations as well as in health food stores and herb shops as essential oil. Never use the seeds or oil internally; they are both toxic.

saged into the scalp, eucalyptus is an effective dandruff treatment.

The oil is widely available commercially, in supermarkets, drug stores, health food stores, and herb shops. The herb is sold as dried leaves, oils, ointments, salves, liniments, and cough drops (in nontoxic doses).

Caution: Despite the practice of some herbalists prescribing small amounts of eucalyptus oil for internal use only, even small doses of the oil can be toxic. Never use eucalyptus oil internally.

SOAPWORT/ BOUNCING BET
(Saponaria officinalis)

One of the best of the "herbal soaps," soapwort—or Bouncing Bet as it is popularly known—has been used at least since the Middle Ages to clean people, animals, and delicate fabrics. In the southern United States, where it was imported by European settlers, it is sometimes called "my lady's washbowl." The root of the plant is saturated with saponins and produces a richly lathering, slightly astringent, soap that is not only a deep skin cleanser—especially for those with large pores and/or oily skin—but also an effective treatment for acne and psoriasis. It may also be used as a dandruff shampoo.

Use soapwort externally for deep cleansing, as an astringent, and in compresses as a treatment for acne and psoriasis. It is available in herb and health food stores as dried and fresh seed, soaps, salves, and oils.

Caution: In the past, folk herbalists prescribed soapwort in small amounts for internal use to treat gout, chest congestion, rheumatism, and venereal disease. However, overdoses of soapwort are toxic and can cause complete muscle paralysis. It should therefore never be taken internally.

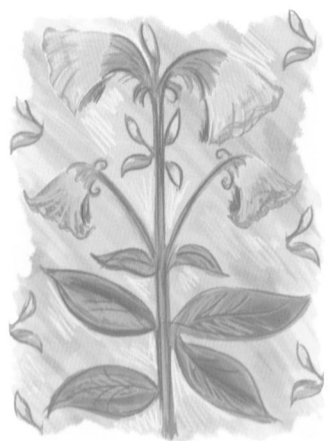

S O A P W O R T /
B O U N C I N G   B E T
(Saponaria officinalis)

As a beauty I'm not a great star,
There are others
more handsome by far;
But my face I don't mind it
Because I'm behind it—
'Tis the folks out in front that I jar.
—ANTHONY EUWER, LIMERATOMY

VERVAIN
(Verbena officinalis, V. hastata)

The large green leaves and small lilac-colored flowers of the vervain plant have been used medicinally in teas and tinctures since at least ancient Greek and Roman times, when the plant was believed to be a

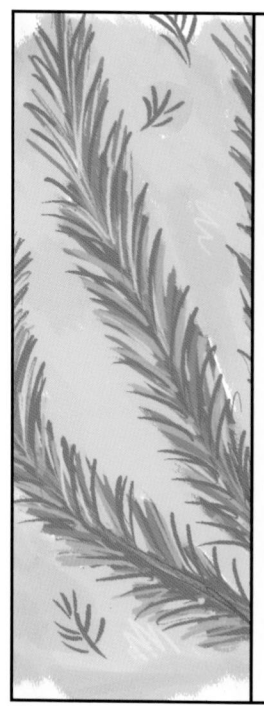

Steamy Brews

FOR THE SKIN

Many herbs can be used as facial steams to deep clean the skin, help remove blackheads, clear up acne, soften dry skin, astringe oily skin, and tighten large pores. Boil one pint of water and pour over two tablespoons of dried herbs which have been placed in a deep bowl or pot; drape a towel over your head (to keep in steam) and place your face about six inches from the container. Steam your face for at least 10 minutes. For general deep cleaning: Use chamomile or rosemary. For blackheads, whiteheads, and acne: Use linden or nettle. For dry skin: Use jojoba or fennel; for oily skin: Use elder or yarrow. For large pores: Use peppermint or horsetail. After steaming, always apply a gentle astringent, such as witch hazel, to close up pores.

---

sacred panacea for every ailment and was commonly called *herba sacra* or *herba veneris*.

Like many of the centuries-old herbs, the use of vervain—also known as herb-of-the-cross (because the crushed flowers were believed to have been used to stop Christ's bleeding)—is steeped in mysticism and magic. Pagans used it as an offering to the gods during their rituals and believed it could confer immortality on its user. Medieval shamans used it to cast love spells, ward off demons, and predict the future.

Not to be confused with the aromatic lemon verbena plant (also called lemon vervain), vervain, sometimes called verbena, was prescribed by early herbalists for everything from the plague to low sex drive, fever, wounds, snake bites, headaches, and jaundice. Today, herbalists most commonly prescribe vervain tea for indigestion, menstrual problems, cystitis, stress, and insomnia. It also relieves pain and swelling and has been used in herbal weight-loss regimens to suppress the appetite. The tea can be taken every day to ease mild stress and

nervousness and used as needed for headaches, toothaches, and sore gums. There is much anecdotal evidence that a strong infusion of the tea, rubbed on the scalp, will promote hair growth.

I don't think of all the misery, but of the beauty that still remains. . . .
My advice is: Go outside, to the fields, enjoy nature and the sunshine, go out and try to recapture happiness in yourself and in God. Think of all the beauty that's still left in and around you and be happy!
—ANNE FRANK,
THE DIARY OF ANNE FRANK

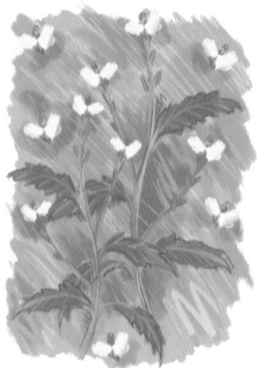

VERVAIN
(Verbena officinalis, V. hastata)

Vervain is available as dried herb, tinctures, decoctions, and tea. No appreciable side effects are associated with its use.

A thing of beauty is a joy for ever;

Its loveliness increases; it will never

Pass into nothingness.

—*JOHN KEATS,*

"ENDYMION I"

Other Helpful Herbs:

■ FOR HEALTHY SKIN: calendula, chamomile, elm, flax, horsetail, strawberry, witch hazel

■ FOR HEALTHY GUMS, MOUTH, AND TEETH: amaranth, echinacea, fennel, parsley, rosemary, sage

■ FOR CELLULITE AND VARICOSE VEINS: butcher's broom, kombucha, milk thistle

■ FOR HEALTHY HAIR: garlic, horsetail

■ FOR HEALTHY EYES: flax, goldenseal

THE A TO Zs OF THE TOP 50 HERBS FOR HEALTH AND HAPPINESS

COMMON ENGLISH NAME	COMMON LATIN NAME	COMMON THERAPEUTIC USES AND ACTIONS	GENERAL DOSAGE INFORMATION
Aloe	*Aloe vera*	Indigestion, gastritis, flatulence, stomach ulcers, burns, wounds, insect bites, sunburn, rashes, poison ivy and poison oak, acne	Follow practitioner's or manufacturer's directions.
Angelica Sinensis, Dong Quai	*Angelica sinensis*	General tonic; menopausal symptoms, PMS, menstrual cramps; anemia, fatigue, poor blood circulation; mild pain reliever and sedative; relief of abscesses, boils, acne, eczema, and psoriasis; angina, high blood pressure	Follow practitioner's or manufacturer's directions.
Arnica	*Arnica montana*	Pain, bruises, springs, inflammations, sports injuries, muscle and joint pain (external use only)	Follow practitioner's or manufacturer's directions. For external use only.
Astragalus	*Astragalus membranaceus*	High blood pressure, fatigue, appetite loss, colds, flu, poor immune system; skin ulcers, acne, boils, hives, eczema, and psoriasis; tissue repair; antibacterial; stimulant	Follow practitioner's or manufacturer's directions. Do not exceed recommended dose.
Barberry	*Berberis vulgaris*	Liver tonic; immune system support; debilitation due to chronic illness; bacterial infections; diarrhea; gallstones; rheumatism; conjunctivitis	Follow practitioner's directions.
Betony	*Stachys officinalis*	Diarrhea; upset stomach, nervous headaches, pain relief, anxiety	Follow practitioner's directions.
Bilberry	*Vaccinium myrtillus*	Gingivitis, mouth sores, varicose veins; eye strain, poor night vision, cataracts, glaucoma Significant antioxidant benefits	Drink 2-3 cups of tea daily.
Black Cohosh	*Cimicifuga racemosa*	General tonic; menopausal symptoms, including hot flashes, depression, night sweat, anxiety, heart palpitations, and vaginal dryness; alternative to conventional estrogen replacement therapy	Follow practitioner's or manufacturer's directions.
Boneset	*Eupatorium perfoliatum*	Fever relief; arthritic, rheumatic, muscle, and joint pain; colds, flu, coughs, upper respiratory congestion	Follow practitioner's directions.
Chamomile, German; Chamomile, Roman	*Matricaria chamomilla; Anthemis nobilis*	Anxiety, stress, insomnia, muscular pain, spasm, and cramps; arthritic joints; burns, wounds, and inflammations	Drink 3-4 cups of tea daily.
Chaste Tree	*Vitex agnus-castus*	Symptoms of premenstrual syndrome (PMS), including bloating, disturbed sleep, tension, anxiety, and mood swings; regulates heavy and irregular periods; mild depression	Follow practitioner's or manufacturer's directions.
Chinese Foxglove Root	*Rehmannia glutinosa*	Blood tonic; nourishes blood, bones, tendons, marrow, eyes, and ears; inhibits effects of aging, including memory loss, senility, and stiff joints; stimulates blood circulation; lowers high blood pressure	Use under practitioner's directions.
Chinese (Club) Moss	*Huperzia serrata*	Contains Huperzine A, a potential treatment for memory loss, learning disabilities, and mental confusion associated with Alzheimer's disease (AD)	Follow practitioner's directions.
Cinnamon Bark	*Cinnamomum verum*	Indigestion; diarrhea; general abdominal discomfort; nausea and vomiting	Follow practitioner's or manufacturer's

Common English Name	Common Latin Name	Common Therapeutic Uses and Actions	General Dosage Information
Cleavers	Galium aparine	Tonsillitis; urinary infections; lymphatic infections; acne, eczema, and psoriasis	Follow practitioner's or manufacturer's directions.
Coltsfoot	Tussilago farfara	Cough suppressant and expectorant; relaxes bronchial tubes; relieves symptoms of asthma and bronchitis	Follow practitioner's directions.
Cramp Bark	Viburnum opulus	Chronic lower back pain; menstrual pain and cramps; muscle spasms; migraines; colic; mild anxiety	Follow practitioner's or manufacturer's directions.
Dandelion	Taraxacum officinale	Water retention; painful and swollen joints; blood, liver, and kidney tonic; helps reduce high blood pressure; relieve edema and other water retention; used for rashes, acne, boils, eczema, poison ivy and poison oak; eliminates warts (externally)	Drink 3-4 cups of tea daily.
Echinacea	Echinacea purpurea, E. angustifolia	Immune stimulant; viral and bacterial infections; colds, flus, bronchitis, ear infections; preventive against cold and flu infections; externally used for boils, abscesses, insect bites, hives, eczema, and cold sores	Follow manufacturer's directions. Available in a variety of forms. Avoid echinacea if you have any type of autoimmune condition.
Elder	Sambucus nigra	Fever relief; immune stimulant; viral and bacterial infections; colds and flu; rich source of vitamins A and C. General antioxidant	Follow practitioner's or manufacturer's directions.
Evening Primrose	Oenothera biennis	Symptoms of premenstrual syndrome (PMS), including bloating, tension, pain, anxiety, and breast pain; anti-inflammatory and anti-clotting properties; also for asthma, whooping cough, colds, arthritis, eczema	Follow practitioner's directions. Consult your physician if you have a blood-clotting disorder.
Eyebright	Euphrasia officinalis	Anti-inflammatory astringent and infection fighter; relieves itchy, red, runny, and irritated eyes	Follow manufacturer's directions.
Feverfew	Tanacetum parthenium	Migraines; pain relief; earache; fever	Follow practitioner's or manufacturer's directions.
Garlic	Allium sativum	Immune stimulant; viral and bacterial infections; colds, flus, coughs; lowers elevated cholesterol levels and reduces high blood pressure; inhibits blood clotting; preventive against atherosclerosis and other forms of heart disease	Follow practitioner's or manufacturer's directions.
Ginger	Zingiber officinale	Nausea, vomiting, motion sickness, indigestion; menstrual cramps; arthritis; colds and flus; lowers elevated cholesterol; inhibits blood clotting	Follow practitioner's or manufacturer's directions. Widely available in a variety of forms.
Ginkgo	Ginkgo biloba	Cerebral and circulatory tonic; dilates blood vessels; prevents blood clotting; increases blood circulation to the brain and heart, and boosts blood-oxygen levels; improves symptoms of mild to moderate mental impairments such as Alzheimer's disease (AD), including poor memory, poor reaction time, and diminished mental acuity; also for colds, allergies, asthma, and arthritis	Follow practitioner's or manufacturer's directions. Do not take if you have a blood-clotting disorder or hemophilia. Do not exceed the minimum recommended doses.

COMMON ENGLISH NAME	COMMON LATIN NAME	COMMON THERAPEUTIC USES AND ACTIONS	GENERAL DOSAGE INFORMATION
Ginseng, Asian	*Panax ginseng*	Greatest of the tonic herbs; reduces mental and physical fatigue; increases mental acuity; strengthens organ functions; heals damage caused by stress; strengthens immune system; normalizes hormone levels	Use under practitioner's directions. Widely available in a variety of forms. Consult practitioner if you have asthma, pressure, heart palpitations, or uterine bleeding.
Green Tea	*Camellia sinensis*	Antioxidant; antibacterial; reduces high cholesterol; lowers high blood pressure; anticlotting properties; preventive against heart disease and cancer. Helps reduce plaque, gingivitis	Drink 3-4 cups daily.
Hawthorn	*Crataegus laevigata, C. oxyacantha*	High blood pressure; blocked arteries; heart palpitations; angina; inflammation of the heart muscle; eases anxiety, stress, and insomnia; strengthens circulatory system and facilitates blood flow; preventive against heart disease	Follow practitioner's or manufacturer's directions. Consult your cardiologist first if you have an existing heart condition.
Kava Kava	*Piper methysticum*	Anxiety, stress, tension; increases mental alertness; relieves insomnia; headaches; muscle spasms and pain; menstrual cramps; arthritic pain; elevates mood; promotes meditative state	Follow practitioner's or manufacturer's directions; do not exceed recommended doses.
Lavender	*Lavandula officinalis*	Stress, tension, depression, anxiety; insomnia; headaches; muscle aches; nausea and flatulence; indigestion; stimulates mental acuity and creativity	Follow practitioner's or manufacturer's directions.
Lemon Balm	*Melissa officinalis*	Irritable bowel syndrome (IBS); stomach and intestinal cramps, spasms, and pain; antibacterial; anxiety, stress, tension; insomnia	Follow practitioner's or manufacturer's directions.
Licorice	*Glycyrrhiza glabra*	Stimulating tonic; raises energy levels; detoxifies the blood; strengthens kidney and spleen function; aids digestion; relieves coughs and diarrhea; regulates appetite and normalizes metabolism	Use under practitioner's directions. Do not use if you have edema, high blood pressure, kidney disease, or glaucoma.
Linden/Lime Blossoms	*Tilia europea*	Preventive and treatment for atherosclerosis and high blood pressure; vasodilating and diuretic effect; anxiety; muscle spasms; stress; colds, coughs, rheumatic pain and sore throats	Follow practitioner's directions. Consult your cardiologist first if you have an existing heart condition.
Marigold/Calendula	*Calendula officinalis*	Bacterial infections; inflammations; bruises, burns, cuts; eczema, acne; stops bleeding; hastens wound-healing	Follow practitioner's directions.
Marshmallow	*Althaea officinalis*	Constipation, gastritis, colitis, and peptic ulcers	Follow manufacturer's directions.
Motherwort	*Leonurus cardiaca*	General heart tonic; stabilizes heart, reduces palpitations, eases pain of angina; relieves muscle spasms and cramping, including menstrual cramping; lowers high blood pressure; relieves edema	Follow practitioner's or manufacturer's directions. Consult your cardiologist first if you have an existing heart condition.
Nettle	*Urtica dioica*	Symptoms of hay fever and general allergy relief. Msy help relieve symptoms associated with prostate enlargement.	Follow manufacturer's directions. Widely availabe in tea form.

COMMON ENGLISH NAME	COMMON LATIN NAME	COMMON THERAPEUTIC USES AND ACTIONS	GENERAL DOSAGE INFORMATION
Peppermint	Mentha piperita	Indigestion, gas, stomach cramps, nausea, motion sickness, insomnia, anxiety, fever, colds and flu	Follow manufacturer's directions.
Plantain Herb Psyllium	Plantago psyllium	Constipation, diarrhea, hemorrhoids, urinary ailments, wound-healing, insect bites, warts	Follow practitioner's or manufacturer's directions. Do not exceed recommended dosage
Red Raspberry	Rubus idaeus	Diarrhea, nausea and vomiting, indigestion	Follow practitioner's or manufacturer's directions.
Rosemary	Rosmarinus officinalis	Complementary therapy for angina, anxiety and stress, muscle spasms and pain. Significant antioxidant benefits	Follow your practitioner's directions. Consult your cardiologist first if you have an existing heart condition.
Sage	Salvia officinalis	Central nervous system tonic, circulatory system tonic, relieves fatigue, exhaustion, and general debilitation associated with prolonged illness, relieves symptoms of depression and severe stress	Drink 3 cups of tea daily as a preventive or follow practitioner's directions. Do not take if you have epilepsy.
Saw Palmetto	Serenoa repens, S. serrulata	Symptoms of benign prostatic hyperplasia (BPH), including increased frequency of urination, burning and pain on urination, reduced force and amount of urine, nighttime urination, difficulty emptying bladder, strengthens genitourinary tract, antiseptic, anti-inflammatory, sedative and diuretic	Use under practitioner's directions.
St. John's Wort	Hypericum perforatum	Best herbal antidepressant, effectively treating the symptoms of mild to moderate depression and seasonal affective disorder (SAD), including sadness, anxiety, low energy, fatigue, irritability, poor concentration, panic attacks, sleep disturbances, and eating disorders	Use under practitioner's directions. Avoid exposure to direct light (sunlight) and always protect eyes and skin.
Valerian	Valeriana officinalis	Insomnia, anxiety, nervous tension, muscle spasms and cramps, pain relief, migraine relief, intestinal pains, menstrual pain	Follow manufacturer's directions. Widely available in a variety of forms. Do not combine with other tranquilizers and sedatives. Do not exceed recommended doses.
Vervain	Verbena officinalis, V. hastata	Indigestion, menstrual problems, cystitis, stress, insomnia, obesity (appetite suppressant), headaches, toothaches and sore gums	Drink up to 3 cups daily.
Wild Yam	Dioscorea villosa	Menstrual cramping and pain, symptoms of menopause, especially hot flashes and irregular, heavy periods	Follow practitioner's directions. Consult physician before using as an estrogen/progesterone supplement.
Wintergreen	Gaultheria procumbens	Pain, inflammations, arthritis and rheumatism, musculoskeletal sprains, spasms, joint and tissue injuries	Follow practitioner's or manufacturer's directions.
Yarrow	Achillea millefolium	Pain, inflammations, wound-healing, backaches, muscular aches and spasms, fever, mildly sedating	Follow practitioner's directions.

Herbal First Aid Kit

The 25 Best Herbal Home Remedies for Cuts, Burns, Insect Bites, Colds, Flu, Coughs, Bronchitis, Sinus Infections, Skin Irritations, Poison Ivy and Poison Oak, Indigestion, Sore Throats, Headaches, Toothaches, Allergies, Nausea, Constipation, Diarrhea, Insomnia, Stress, and Anxiety.

No herbal first aid kit should be without these 25 super healing herbs. All are readily available, in a variety of forms, at health food stores, herb shops, herbal pharmacies, and drug stores. Keep all herbs in their original containers and store them in a dark, cool place. For more information about each herb, see the individual herb entries throughout the book.

- **ALOE:** externally for insect bites, bee stings, minor burns, chapped skin, and sunburn
- **CALENDULA:** externally for chapped skin, rashes, minor cuts and bruises, and insect bites
- **CHAMOMILE:** internally for indigestion, insomnia, colic, and mild anxiety
- **CHASTE TREE:** internally for PMS
- **CLOVE:** externally for toothaches
- **CRAMP BARK:** internally for menstrual cramps
- **DANDELION:** internally as a mild restorative and diuretic
- **ECHINACEA:** internally for colds, flu, sore throat, bronchitis, and sinus infections
- **ELDER:** internally for fevers
- **EYEBRIGHT:** internally and externally for strained, tired, and irritated eyes
- **FEVERFEW:** internally for headaches
- **GARLIC:** externally for ear infections; internally for bacterial infections
- **GINGER:** internally as a mild restorative and for indigestion, gas, fatigue, and nausea
- **KAVA:** internally for anxiety, stress, and insomnia
- **LEMON BALM:** internally for irritable bowel syndrome and indigestion
- **MARSHMALLOW:** internally for cystitis and other bladder infections
- **NETTLE:** internally for allergies
- **PEPPERMINT:** internally for indigestion, migraine headaches, and diarrhea
- **PLANTAIN:** externally for poison ivy and poison oak
- **PSYLLIUM:** internally for constipation
- **SAGE:** internally for sore throats and sinus infections
- **TEA TREE:** externally for fungus infections, including athlete's foot
- **VALERIAN:** internally for mild anxiety, menstrual cramps, and insomnia
- **WITCH HAZEL:** externally for rashes, itching, poison ivy, poison oak, tired eyes, and hemorrhoids
- **YARROW:** internally for pain